# LET ME LISTEN TO YOUR HEART

# LET ME LISTEN TO YOUR HEART

## Writings by Medical Students

♥

Edited by David S. Svahn, M.D.
Collected by Alan J. Kozak, M.D.


Foreword by Frank Davidoff, M.D.
Editor Emeritus, *Annals of Internal Medicine*

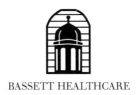

BASSETT HEALTHCARE

BOOK PRODUCTION

*Executive Editor*: David S. Svahn
*Editorial Consultant*: Valerie Tomaselli
*Production Consultant*: Chris Moschovitis
*Administrative Assistants*: Sue Garvin, Leann Smith
*Copy Editor*: Carole Campbell
*Design and Layout*: Annemarie Redmond
*Cover Design*: Dan Jock, Jayson Tillapaugh
*Printing*: Carr Printing, Endwell, N.Y.


BASSETT HEALTHCARE HUMANITIES AND MEDICINE PROGRAM

*Developers*: Alan J. Kozak, Michael Foltzer
*Coordinator*: David S. Svahn


BASSETT HEALTHCARE OFFICE OF MEDICAL EDUCATION

*Director*: Walter Franck
*Internal Medicine Medical Student Course Director*: Alan J. Kozak

Made possible in part through a grant from the Arnold P. Gold Foundation
Second Printing

# THANK YOU

*Robin Ackerman*

Intimate details
of your life
of your body
you share with me.

The white coat
the title "medical student"
the stethoscope
open the door.

You came to see the doctor
yet you allow me
to educate myself
at your expense.

Who am I
to receive
this honor
this respect?

I will be
forever indebted
to your generosity
Thank You.

# CONTENTS

# FOREWORD

*Frank Davidoff, M.D.*

Doctors, being people, are just like everyone else; at the same time, doctors are different—very different. What's more, the process by which ordinary people are transformed into doctors is mysterious, even to those going through it, more so to those outside medicine. First, during their training doctors enter into a conceptual world that's vastly different from most people's. The myriad mental models that make up that world—complex, intricate models of structure, and function, and causality—are the result of hundreds of years of probing into human biology and behavior, countless person-years of thought, thousands of observations and experiments. The models are both abstract (you can't see most of the things they describe—for example, who has actually seen a blood sugar?) and practical (they have great, albeit imperfect, power to predict risk, define illness, decide on treatment).[1]

Second, during their training doctors have privileged experiences; they see and hear things allowed to only a few: patients' deepest fears and darkest secrets; the great and mysterious events of life: life-threatening illness, grievous loss, birth, death. It has been pointed out, for example, that the only people who have contact with more dead bodies than doctors do are soldiers in wartime. A non-medical friend of Eric Michael David, one of the students who writes in this volume, put it this way, in discussing David's experience of dissecting a cadaver: "You know what the difference is between doctors and everyone else? Doctors have seen what's on the other side of the bellybutton. What the heck is back there? Does it lead into my stomach? Is it connected to some sort of tube? Is there a tiny little knot tied in the back? We don't know! But you've seen what's back there. To have that demystified fundamentally changes you with respect to everyone else."[2]

During their training doctors are tested against punishing standards of performance. Even in their pre-medical studies they're required to master (and remember) huge amounts of scientific and technical information; during medical school the demands are even greater. But although knowing a lot is necessary, it isn't sufficient. Doctors also need to do things, and do them extremely well, or else— extreme demands are hardly unique to doctoring, but there's a lot at stake here; medical mistakes cause pain, and suffering, and death. During their clinical training, medical students and residents are required to learn many difficult and demanding things: to do delicate and potentially dangerous invasive procedures like spinal taps and threading catheters into the heart; to make complex decisions, often very fast, and under conditions of great uncertainty; and to work almost inhuman hours, often in the face of "sleeplessness, isolation from the outside world, impairment of social relationships, poor diet, frequent patient presentations, lectures and seminars, and relentless cross-examination by superiors about everything."[3]

Why does medical education cling to such extreme traditions? Reflecting on his own medical training, the anthropologist Melvin Konner considers a number of practical and historical reasons, but ends up suggesting a deeper explanation: "The risks and the pain are what give you the power to heal. As a sometime apprentice in both systems— the !Kung [a tribe of African bushmen] and the American—I can say that the confidence to heal comes in part through the pain; that you feel justified in exercising such terrible power over your fellow human beings to the extent that you have suffered to get the power; and, last but not least, your patients feel it too."[3] This is a strong statement. But does medical training really need to be so grueling? Or is Konner's explanation one way that those who have gone through a harsh, painful experience justify it to themselves and the rest of the world? And, as Konner himself notes, could such experiences even contribute to doctors' widely-perceived tendency to distance themselves from their patients?

A substantial and growing literature is emerging on the experience of doctoring, including the "On Being a Doctor" section of *Annals of Internal Medicine*,[4] but with a few exceptions (such as Konner's account), relatively little literature exists on the strange transformative experiences of medical training. It was therefore a particular pleasure during my tenure as editor of *Annals* to learn from David Svahn about the medical student-writing project in Cooperstown that has led to publication of this book. At one point he and I even discussed the possibility of starting a new section in *Annals* called "On Becoming a Doctor." Although for a variety of reasons that wasn't possible, our discussions did introduce me to a unique program and a unique body of written work.

The pieces in this volume are not experiences reflected on in tranquility, long after the fact; they were written on the spot. Indeed, a large part of their uniqueness lies in the freshness and immediacy that comes with this sort of you-had-to-be-there reports from "the trenches."

Perhaps more important, they are unique because they successfully get past the technical and professional, and go on into the human dimension of medicine; into students' first experience of walking the fine line between getting close enough to your patients to see them as people, and staying detached enough from them to be medically effective; into the reflection and self-revelation that come with intense personal growth. Ultimately, it's reassuring to know that although medical training is in many ways irrational and extreme, at its best (as it appears to be in Cooperstown) learning medicine can be, and is, a humanizing experience. So read these accounts, and be instructed; be amazed; and be comforted—be very comforted.

[1] F. Davidoff, "Who Has Seen a Blood Sugar? The Shaping of the Invisible World." In *Who Has Seen a Blood Sugar? Reflections on Medical Education* (Philadelphia: American College of Physicians, 1996): 96–100.

[2] E. M. David, "Thoughts from Gross Anatomy," *Annals of Internal Medicine* 131 (1999): 974–5.

[3] M. Konner, *Becoming a Doctor: A Journey of Initiation in Medical School* (New York: Viking Penguin, 1987): 371–4.

[4] M. A. LaCombe, ed. *On Being a Doctor 2. Voices of Physicians and Patients* (Philadelphia: American College of Physicians, 2000).

# PREFACE

*Let Me Listen to Your Heart* presents some of the best writing by third-year medical students over a period of six years at The Mary Imogene Bassett Hospital in Cooperstown, New York. The students are required to write as part of their training in primary care medicine at the several clinics that constitute Bassett Healthcare.

The book begins with a Foreword by Frank Davidoff, M.D., editor emeritus of the *Annals of Internal Medicine*. His reflections on the nature of medical practice and the training of physicians provide a vital and contemplative touchstone for the writings that make up the body of the book. The Introduction explains the rationale for incorporating humanities into the training of physicians and describes the development of the Bassett program. The writings that follow are grouped into thematic chapters, although it should be noted that, just as the experience of the medical students is complex and multifaceted, the themes chosen to organize the material are impressionistic and overlapping rather than definitive. Recognizing that some of our readers will be interested in looking more into the use of the humanities in medicine, we have provided a Reading List of selected journals at the end of the book.

We were guided through the publication process by the patient, friendly, and professional advice of Valerie Tomaselli and Chris Moschovitis of The Moschovitis Group. Our thanks to Leann Smith and Sue Garvin for administrative support. Constructive criticism was provided by Pat Dillon, Rita Ferrandino, Tom Milligan, Karin Svahn and Michael Willis. We are particularly indebted to Frank Davidoff, Marilyn Wesley, and Carol Frost, superb writers and teachers, for in-depth review and criticism. Rita Charon's encouragement for this and related endeavors has helped keep us moving. The story "Sinusitis" by Eric David, written for our program, has been accepted for publication in the *Annals of Internal Medicine*; we gratefully acknowledge the editor's permission to include it here. We acknowledge the devotion to teaching of the many Bassett physicians who act as preceptors for the students and, finally, we express our thanks and admiration to all the students, published or not, who have written so enthusiastically and movingly about their work.

We hope the reader finds these pieces as inspiring as we have. They are presented as written with minor changes in names and some details in an effort to preserve anonymity. With the support of Bassett's Medical Education Endowment Fund and a generous grant from the Arnold P. Gold Foundation we publish this work in order to share, with Bassett staff, alumni, and friends, and a larger public, the remarkable feelings and acute awareness of our fine doctors-in-training. We believe such a program may be used anywhere there are dedicated students and teachers and hope that this book inspires others to do similar work.

Inquiries and comments about content are welcome and may be directed to David Svahn, at Bassett Healthcare, One Atwell Road, Cooperstown, New York 13326 or dsvahn@stny.rr.com. Inquiries regarding purchase of copies may be directed to the Office of Medical Education, Bassett Healthcare, One Atwell Road, Cooperstown, N.Y. 13326 or medical.education@bassett.org. Income from sales will accrue to Bassett's Medical Education Endowment Fund in support of the Humanities and Medicine Program.

# INTRODUCTION

*David S. Svahn, M.D.*

*The first staggering fact about medical education is that after two . . .
years of being taught on the assumption that everyone is the same, the
student has to find out for himself that everyone is different . . .*

—Robert Platt (*British Medical Journal*, 1965)

## BECOMING A PHYSICIAN AND THE ROLE OF WRITING

Becoming a physician is not easy. It takes time to learn the requisite
facts and skill to develop ability in communication. The awarding of
the M.D. degree after four years of school is followed by further training as a "resident" physician for several years—a long and arduous yet
exhilarating process. As one of our contributors, Erica Shoemaker, put
it, writing from the vantage point of several years of post-graduate
training, the process "seems too short and endlessly long, a burden and
welcome perfection, all at the same time."

There have been important developments in medical education in
the past several decades. Among them, George Engel's biopsychosocial
model of medicine has gradually gained acceptance.[1] It teaches the
importance of the psychological and social aspects of illness in addition to the biological. Then, primary care medicine has achieved
recognition as a field demanding special skills and training, hence the
introduction of primary care tracks in residency programs and primary care rotations for students in the third or fourth year of medical
school.[2] Primary care physicians are trained broadly in internal medi-

cine and family medicine programs to interpret and manage a wide variety of concerns; they are the modern general practitioners who learn to appreciate that all aspects of their patients' lives are relevant to their health.

A major development is the concept that formal teaching of the humanities—including literary studies—need not, indeed should not, stop with admission to medical school. It has been thought for two decades or more that physicians will benefit professionally by reading literature and writing creatively. Scholars Rita Charon,[3] Anne Hunsaker Hawkins,[4] and Kathryn Montgomery Hunter[5] are among those who currently teach humanities on medical school faculties and write extensively about literature and medicine in journals and books devoted to the link between the two fields. Traditional medical journals now regularly include creative writing and essays about the human side of medicine.

How does the study of literature benefit physicians? Not simply valuable as entertainment, literary study is useful professionally. It encourages lucid presentation of narrative, requiring physicians to listen to their patients' often complex stories. In an increasingly technical world, the importance, both in diagnosis and treatment, of simply listening to the patient tell his story needs reinforcement.

## WRITING BY STUDENTS

For medical students, with one foot in the lay world and one in the professional, literary activity is helpful in several ways. First, literature helps to legitimize the validity of feelings in the practice of medicine. Then, literature deals with conflict, ambiguity, and uncertainty—a focus that contrasts with the reductionist nature of science. The practice of medicine involves both art and science and literary study helps students achieve the balance required in the skilled practitioner. Students enter medical school familiar with their own feelings, uncertainty, and life stories. Literary study during school and later helps keep them in touch with these feelings and to value the feelings and stories of their patients; in short, it helps to maintain the humanism that brought them to medicine in the first place.

In 1996 Dr. Alan Kozak, Internal Medicine Medical Student Course Director at The Mary Imogene Bassett Hospital in Cooperstown, New York, initiated a requirement for third-year students taking their primary care clerkships to write a poem, story, or essay reflecting on their experiences in learning to care for patients.

Inspired by the humanistic mentoring of Dr. George Engel during his own education at the University of Rochester, Dr. Kozak wished to encourage the expression and sharing of insights and feelings about the learning and practice of medicine, feelings that might not otherwise be openly discussed—the insecurity, fear, satisfaction, and awe— as students begin to work with patients. It works. In sharing their reflections, they learn to know their patients, their colleagues, and themselves better. The writing has often been remarkable in a literary sense and in depth of feeling, sometimes in both qualities. *Let Me Listen to Your Heart* is a collection of the best of the students' work.

The themes of this writing are as difficult to categorize as are the patients themselves, which is indeed one of the challenges students face in learning to practice the profession. Some work deals with the uncertainty inherent in clinical medicine, the frustration in finding that the illness of individuals is not, as textbooks often suggest, clearcut. Many stories and poems deal with old age and dying and how patients and families cope. Some describe the insecurities endemic among medical students; other pieces reaffirm their choice of profession. A common theme is the exhilaration and satisfaction at being intimately involved in patients' lives, of bonding, of being able to help, of making a difference. Many describe individual patients who strike a personal chord, reminding the students of people they've known, of family members. Some write of facing their own inevitable aging and illness. Not a few write about the thrill of making that first correct diagnosis, of receiving thanks or a pat on the back from a mentor or an appreciative patient. They write about learning that listening is both diagnostic and therapeutic and that touch is a powerful tool.

The physicians-in-training who have written this collection are of varied ethnic, demographic, educational and socio-economic backgrounds. Some plan to pursue primary care internal medicine as a career; others will train as medical or surgical sub-specialists. What unites the writers is their level of clinical inexperience; they are all third-year students reflecting on their earliest in-depth experiences with sick people in an out-patient setting. Except for one half-day per week for classroom teaching and discussion with the course director, the students' time during their Bassett primary care rotation is spent with their teachers—all experienced practicing clinicians. Although the students work primarily in the office setting, some physicians take their students along on house calls, and to see patients at local nursing homes, jails, and other venues The experiences at the root of this collection vary widely and so do the stories based on them.

## THE TRANSITION FROM CLASSROOM TO CLINIC

The medical school experience is roughly divided into two periods with training in the classroom and laboratory during the first two years followed by clinical training in hospitals, clinics, and practitioners' offices. Though many schools introduce students to patients in a minor way as early as the first year, the students seldom have a real sense of involvement and responsibility for patients before the third year. The shift in basic science concepts and models to those of the clinic is a major change and stress as students begin to apply what they have learned in the classroom to patients. Even the vocabulary and reasoning skills of clinical work are new.[6] Thus, a significant transition occurs as students move into the third year. Further, the students find, as they begin to work with patients, that the facts in their textbooks and lecture notes are of little use without a well-developed ability to interview patients and to understand their concerns. They find that though they know disease in detail, they need to learn to understand illness—the individual's experience of disease. To know who the patients are is just as important as how they are.

## WRITING AND THE HEART

We not only think that writing about their experiences helps students grow in skill and insight, but also believe that the general public may appreciate and benefit from these stories. There is a broad interest in medicine and in the insights into human nature that medical situations and relationships offer. The writing is both inspiring and reassuring. For a public suspicious that physicians are losing their humanity in a technical age, these pieces offer reassurance. They show that our students are learning to listen to their patients and that they are touched by the depth of human suffering and the heights of hope they encounter. One may ask if this is representative of all students. Although our writings are by a relatively few we think it likely that most, if not all, students similarly exposed to experienced practitioners will gain the same insights.

The medical examination of the heart requires a certain physical intimacy and physicians may announce to patients their wish to do this with a statement such as "Let me listen to your heart." For these stories and poems about students getting to know patients as well as themselves, it seems an appropriate title.

[1] G. Engel, "The Need for a New Medical Model: A Challenge for Biomedicine," *Science* 196 (1977): 129–36.

[2] E. Cassell, *Doctoring: The Nature of Primary Care Medicine* (New York: Oxford University Press, 1997).

[3] R. Charon, "Literature and Medicine: Origins and Destinies," *Academic Medicine* 75 (2000): 23–7.

[4] A. H. Hawkins and M. C. McIntyre, eds. *Teaching Literature and Medicine* (New York: The Modern Language Association, 2000).

5 K. M. Hunter, *Doctors' Stories: The Narrative Structure of Medical Knowledge* (Princeton, N.J.: Princeton University Press, 1991).

6 H. G. Schmidt, G. R. Norman, and H. P. Boshuizen, "A Cognitive Perspective on Medical Expertise: Theory and Implications," *Academic Medicine* 65 (1990): 611–21.

CHAPTER ONE

# Insecurity & Affirmation

♥

*In learning to talk to his patients, the doctor may*
*talk himself back into loving his work. He has little to lose and*
*everything to gain by letting the sick man into his heart.*

—Anatole Broyard (*Intoxicated by My Illness*, 1997)

When students move on from the preclinical period of medical school—when they leave the classroom for the examining room—they are usually both exhilarated and terrified. "This is it," they think at first, "this is what it's all about. This is what I really want to do, what I endured biochemistry for, to see patients, make diagnoses, assist at surgery, maybe save a life." But then comes the doubt, the lack of confidence, described by Kathryn Montgomery Hunter as ". . . the appalling moment at the beginning of clinical training when [students] are compelled to realize that, despite their years of successful study in the basic sciences, they know next to nothing that would be of any help to a patient."

Students' personal insecurity, aggravated by the uncertainty inherent in all of medicine, often leads to doubts about their ability and even about their choice of profession. Invariably, at some point in their training they will experience the satisfaction of realizing they can help patients simply by taking the time to listen. At other times he or she will receive praise from a teacher or, most gratifyingly, thanks from a patient. These are often defining moments in a student's professional development and, in some cases, powerfully reaffirm the original motivation to study medicine. The following stories represent this range of feeling—from doubt and insecurity to satisfaction and affirmation.

# HEALING HANDS

*Livia Santiago-Rosado*

She said, at first, she wanted to heal.
Like her great-grandmother before her
a healer of body and soul with
a well-meant word and a well-placed hand.
But then there was the problem of the
equations and the formulas of total peripheral
resistance. And the Wenckebachs, the Reiters, the
continuing Chiaris, the minutiae of von Recklinghausens,
the Creutzfelds and the Jakobs. A-line, BMs, C-pap,
hepatitidies, vasculitidies, viral gastroenteritidies, mysterious
mitochondrial heredities. A syringe for a syrinx, some injection in
the throat, toxic shock from tamponade? Snap
or crackles in the lung fields, copper
wiring in the eye grounds, is it pacing or a gallop.
There were crypts and there were villi,
fluid flagella, powerful pili conspiring in the
seemingly exponential pharmacokinetic elimination of
knowledge, the infratherapeutic level of fact.
Fibrillation versus flutter, leiomyoma or myosarcoma,
was it obstructive or restrictive, this alkalotic acidemia of
detail and disease.

In the middle was Ms. S, skeptical, guarding
with her gaze. What is she, this little girl, inferring
from my pain? Will she hurt me even more with her
inexperienced hand, will she download memories with
her fancy probing tongue, will she talk me half to
death, and then leave me there to scorch? Where's a doctor,

or a nurse, for heaven's sake an orderly? Get me a
receptionist, for God's sake, let me sigh and writhe in peace. Then
her own voice, silent whisper quivering in insecurity,
shivering in inadequacy, clamoring for
accuracy or at the least a brain. Please, to remember something
in the differential, the guidelines and the regimens,
some diagnostic acumen, and first to do no harm. Please, to
listen to the COPD's lung, the IBD's abdomen, to check the RA's ESR.

But then at last was Mr. D who came in with a bad back. Toiling
daily with his cattle, over sixty years, untiring
raised four children and a barn. So they talked about the City, and the
village politicians, shared a laugh about the season, she learned all about
his farm. She then taught about stenosis, nerve compression and necrosis,
hypothesized about neuritis, or a touch of mild arthritis,
but not in so many words.
Sent him, recommended rest, and proudly sporting his prescription,
he shook her hand so long. In the end, just two weeks later,
smiling friendly Mr. D came to thank her for the cure. He was
better, back was painless, he was going back to work. She told him
she milked a cow, and the farmer grinned with glee,
and they shared another laugh but her
eye began to tear when he said you cured me, doc. I think I am healed.
And she smiled and said good luck, and once more now more secure
she shook his hand.

❤

# ON SEEING TWO DEER IN THE WOODS

*Matthew Salomone*

On seeing two deer in the woods . . .

> I approach them,
> I am not seen, but existence known.
> Their ears twitch
> with each step I am closer,
>> closer to them,
>>> closer to me.

> unsure of myself,
>> unsure of my footing,
> if I miss-step will they run?

> Into view from between the wood
>> sunlight illuminating my crown
> breaking their darkness into my world.
> They glance with quizzical stares,
>> as if I know;
> as if I have the answers
>> to the world,
>>> to everything,
>>>> to this place.

> Their muscles quiver with fear!
> (or am I the one shaking?)
> close enough to touch them;
>> close enough to hear their labored breaths
> and feel their warmth against my own,

Yet I pull back,
    Not ready.
and frightened by their being;
frightened by what lies beyond their coat,
    I dare not disturb.
For their skin is like my own.
    I pause,
        I fumble,
           and . . .

They understand.
I mean no harm
just curiosity driving me closer
    until they take flight
        and are gone . . .

# GETTING THROUGH

*Corey Magnell*

"So how are you today?"

What a stupid, stupid question. I know how you are—sick of freshmen like me practically giddy from my expensive education. You've seen me before. Clones just like me have barged into your room and gaped at your half-dissected neck, curious as to what half a tongue looks like. You think I can't take my eyes off your skin, raw and scaling from your chin to your nipples—your reward for months spent under a radiation beam. You don't want to have anything to do with me and my college-educated, city-girl, manicured enthusiasm. I disgust you.

But still, why don't you answer me?

You look weary when I ask you to open your mouth, as you've done so many times since that spot appeared under your tongue and nearly ate it away. Why do I need to see inside, I'm sure you're asking yourself, when there's nothing left to see but the stump of my tongue? Have a look, everybody else has. You startle and jump a full two inches off the table when I reach out to touch your neck.

"Does it hurt?"

"No."

"Does it itch?"

"No."

"Does it bother you?"

A shrug.

I can see you stiffening up, getting ready for the usual lecture on smoking and boozing. You've been told so many times that your cancer is the price one pays for the years of cigarettes and liquor. But I'm sure the guilt pierces deeper than that. That you find it hard to fathom that something so simple and pleasurable such as a smoke could do something so horrible, so painful. There has to be another reason. No, I think I'll spare you the tobacco diatribe today. You've heard it too many times. Besides, what would I do in your place?

At a loss for what to do next, I begin a review of systems, the lazy man's guide to conversation.

"How's your appetite?"

"Terrible."

"How are you sleeping?"

"All day."

"How's your mood?"

Another shrug.

Is this my best attempt at empathy? I, who promised myself I wouldn't become one of those doctors who trample over the sick with callousness. I, who wanted to grow old with my patients, hear about the weddings, the school recitals, the retirement plans. I, who never wanted to fear my patients' illnesses or despairs. This was all my "bedside manner" could muster?

But I knew this man could see right through me. That he would smirk at my feeble efforts to reach out. My stomach twisted with nausea as I stepped forward.

"You know, there's so much we can do for you to make you feel better. There's no reason you should spend all day in bed. Have you ever thought about talking to someone, getting this out of your system?"

You look away and stare passively at the scale across the room. I have to go on, although I already know the answer to my next question.

"Would you be interested in taking something which might get you out of bed, help you cope with things?"

You pick at a ragged spot on your jeans. I begin to reel from the overwhelming odor of cigarette smoke on your clothing which makes my anxiety even more unbearable.

But then you look up and fixate on my shoulder.

"Yes."

# TIRED

*Josette Rivera*

After the last harrowing inpatient rotation, I was tired. If I had had enough energy, I probably would have felt desperate to get away from it all—from the hospital, from the medical school, from everything. As luck would have it, my name was pulled out of a hat, and I got the coveted Cooperstown rotation. I arrived with an intense hope that somehow my spirit, my curiosity, and my attitude toward medicine would change for the better.

Pervasive changes occurred almost immediately after I moved, as I now had time to think, study, and sleep. I never previously considered myself to be an "outdoors" person, but since living in Cooperstown, I always want to be outside. My favorite find is a place at Lake Otsego where you can sit within a small clearing at the water's edge, and the trees grant some privacy. One Sunday afternoon there, as I was caught up in a moment of brilliant sunlight, autumn colors, and silence, I realized that the core of my problem was a feeling of guilt for being so unmotivated about medicine.

This, too, changed while working at a small rural clinic in one of New York's poorest counties. As one might expect from national statistics, patients with diabetes, chronic lung disease, depression, and anxiety filled the schedule almost daily. Yet in the midst of socio-economic depression were unforgettable examples of self-reliance, inner strength, and optimism, especially among some chronically ill patients who had defied death on multiple occasions. The lady at the minimart across the street from the clinic said that news spreads quickly in their tiny village, and the word was "That doctor is a good one, easy to talk to." My impression was that since my preceptor had begun working at the clinic, many people in the region, including those who hadn't been to a doctor for years, had started coming to the clinic, and sometimes for no other reason than curiosity.

My preceptor was a young doctor with keen intelligence, insight, and wit. I was impressed by how he thoughtfully addressed his patients' concerns. He knew when to talk and when to just listen. He made decisions based on a blend of evidence-based medicine and common sense. Whenever he left me alone with patients, they would often tell me, "You're lucky you're working with a great doctor. Yep, we really like him." Their faces revealed a deep appreciation and respect. He remembered the trials of being a medical student and made teaching a priority. And somehow, we had time to talk about politics, his carnival glass collection, and "the kids these days." I showed him how to say "Ay caramba!" after seeing difficult patients. I loved going to work every day because I knew that I would learn and have fun in the process.

Looking back, I realize that, prior to this experience, I had lost my sense of purpose, generating a sense of guilt and alienation from my classmates. Watching my preceptor with his patients helped me to answer the question, "Why am I doing this?" which had entered my often sleep-deprived mind. In the process of observing his skill as a physician and teacher, I lost the guilt and regained my enthusiasm.

♥

## FRIDAY AFTERNOON

*Colleen Barber*

It was a dreary Friday afternoon, 3 P.M., last appointment of the day. I glanced quickly at the schedule and it looked as though the last patient was here for a nursing home medicine check. I looked over at my attending as he said, ". . . not sure what she's here for, it seems like she always has some vague complaint that we can't fix." This didn't sound like a particularly satisfying way to end the week. Flipping through the chart I got a quick gestalt of what the attending was alluding to as I scanned pages of multiple visits for unresolved somatic complaints—low back pain, chronic abdominal pain, constipation, etc. The medication list was even less reassuring as the entire page was filled with numerous medications that had been prescribed futilely in an attempt to provide some relief.

I knocked quickly on the door, walked in, and introduced myself as I've done many times before—"Hello, my name is Colleen, I'm a medical student working with Dr. X today. Nice to meet you," I said almost reflexively, expecting the usual smile or nod. Instead, I was abruptly greeted with the words, "Oh, I didn't want to see you." Jokingly I replied, "Well, you have to since I'm already here." "No, I don't have to do anything," said the eighty-something, tiny, gray-haired woman seated on the exam table, fully clothed, clutching her handbag. Quickly I realized that this woman was indeed very serious. "Well, that's true," I replied, "I could go outside and wait for Dr. X to see you but he won't be in for while." There was a moment of silence that seemed to say to me that I should attempt to stay and talk, because there was clearly something more on her agenda than a medicine check.

I decided that my usual opening line, the standard, "So, what brings you to the office today," was not going to work with this patient who was less than excited to see me as it was. I decided that I was better off addressing some of her prior concerns so that she would think that I was abreast of her care and possibly feel more comfortable talking with me.

"How has your abdominal pain been lately?" "Terrible," she replied. "What about your back?" "Terrible," she again replied. "What do you mean 'terrible'?" I said. "Terrible, you know, no better, that's what I mean. So bad that I just wish I could jump in the lake and die." Suddenly, I was beginning to get very concerned about this woman, wishing she would open up to me.

Desperate for words, I attempted to continue the conversation by asking her if anything had improved since her last visit six weeks ago. "I don't know, you ask me about something and I'll tell you," she replied. Considering there was really nothing else specifically detailed in the chart, it didn't look like I was going to get very far. I needed another strategy and soon, or else she was sure to kick me out of the room for wasting her time. I decided to pursue her earlier comment about being dead by searching for other signs of depression. She assured me that she was sleeping like a baby, in fact she as sleeping so well that she didn't seem to ever want to get out of bed. She was not eating much, but that was because of the quality of the food at the "home." The home? I had almost forgotten that she was a nursing home resident. The food is so bad, she told me that people downtown are always laughing and joking about what they feed "them" at the home. Her puffy swollen eyes and long face prompted me to ask her when she last felt happy.

It was like a dam breaking loose, as her eyes filled with tears and she began to sob. "It was before she was sent to the home," she confided. I encouraged her to tell me more about what was making her so sad. Over the next 30 minutes she proceeded to tell me how she used to live with her younger sister until two years ago when she died of cancer. She then moved in with her older sister, who soon had a stroke and was put into the home. It was then that she, herself, went to the home to be closer to her sister. Apparently that didn't last long because her sister was moved to a higher level of care in Pennsylvania. "I just miss them so much," she said, "everyone I love is gone." She continued on to explain how her baby brother had just died six months ago and that now she felt as though she had no one left. I asked her about friends at the home and she told me about her best girlfriend at the home who had become "too big for her britches," and this had caused a falling-out between them. Tears streamed down her face as she recalled her numerous attempts at mending the friendship. As she paused, I told her that I should probably bring Dr. X in to join the conversation so that we could discuss ways to help decrease her sadness. She nodded, but told me that she didn't think there was anything that could possibly help at this point.

Dr. X soon arrived and joined in the discussion. "How come you haven't told me how you have been feeling?" he said. "Because you didn't ask," she replied. She looked fondly over toward me and acknowledged that I had asked the right questions. She lamented her losses once again, as I held her hand, patted her back, and passed her tissues. The box of tissues was gone by the time we finished discussing everything and decided to try a new medicine similar to the antidepressant she had taken in the past.

After Dr. X left I stayed and went over her medication list with her once again, carefully writing all the adjustments down for her to take back to the home. She tried to joke sarcastically with me about being a crazy old woman and I reassured her that she was in no way crazy. She was simply reacting to a lot of sad circumstances and the loss of many very special people. She nodded and quickly changed the subject to her wheelchair, which she needed for travel back to the home. For some reason I felt as though I should be the one to wheel her out to the waiting room and see her through the end of her visit. I needed closure . . . I didn't want her to think that I had quickly forgotten her sorrows and moved on to the next patient. As we arrived in the waiting area, she turned to me and told me that she loved me and was very thankful for all I had done for her.

I realized at that moment that my role as a medical student is a very sacred one. An hour before I was thinking about how frustrating it is to listen to multiple complaints that have been addressed time and time again, and now I was feeling quite satisfied with myself for offering a fresh perspective. I am convinced that I made a difference in this patient's life simply by listening and truly hearing what she was trying to tell us all along.

♥

# Rewards

*Clarissa Bonanno*

I stepped out of the room to take a deep breath. Walking over to the nurse's station I tried to keep my expression from revealing my frustration. Before organizing my notes from a particularly scattered encounter with a patient, I said quietly, as lightheartedly as I could manage, "It's just not like it is in the books . . . " I was referring to the patient's multiple vague complaints which I had no idea how to assess or interrelate. One of the young physician assistants, whose preternatural wisdom I had already come to appreciate, said cheerfully, "But that's why you went into this, right?" In case he was presuming that I would be nothing but intrigued by a diagnostic challenge, I didn't want to disappoint him. "Yes," I replied, "I suppose so." In reality, I was merely frustrated.

Earlier in the year, on the final day of my psychiatry rotation, my preceptor presented me with an article and some final words of advice. Despite spending almost five weeks working together, I had not come to know him well. He possessed the psychiatrist's inclination to conceal completely his own thoughts and opinions. Thus his parting words took on a distinct significance. He said, "Read this once in a while. Medicine, you will find, is a difficult field. Try, if you can, to remember why you went into it and keep that with you." The article was a reflection written by a medical school admissions committee member. He wrote that after many years of perusing essays citing the applicant's love of science as the inspiration for a career in medicine, he was still waiting for the first candidate to propose that love of human beings had been the motivation.

This memory has remained a disquieting one for me. I have always felt it was my interest in science that led me to medicine. There is something almost mysteriously fascinating about human disease. Perhaps it is that these problems illuminate how elegantly composed life, particularly human life, is. Of course, the ultimate goal of using medical knowledge to help people live longer and healthier lives has always been of prime importance to me. But somehow, this year, while my depth of clinical knowledge has expanded, my understanding of pathophysiology has begun to fade, and I have found myself missing that simplicity, that elegance.

My next patient that day was an 85-year-old woman who was coming in for follow-up of her hypertension and hypothyroidism. The visit appeared a fairly routine one, so in the interest of time I did not review the whole of her chart. I entered the room and introduced myself, inquiring if the patient would mind seeing a medical student. The nurses usually ask the patient beforehand, but I have made a habit of doing so, if only for a place to begin each time. The patient, Mrs. Arnold, said, "Well, what would you do if I said I did?" in a tone that told me her mind remained as sharp as her sense of humor. I also learned that she enjoys being physically active, swimming at the local sports center three times per week—"Just this morning. That's why my hair looks so lovely."—and walking regularly with a friend. Though her friend "only strolls," Mrs. Arnold is glad for the company.

When my preceptor came in she rounded out Mrs. Arnold's extensive medical history for me. Several years ago she was severely debilitated by osteopenia. She was so severely affected, in fact, that an extensive workup was initiated for a neoplastic process underlying her condition. Over the following years an amelanotic melanoma and then a breast cancer were diagnosed. Both were treated surgically, without resolution of disease. Finally, the workup of a deep vein thrombosis revealed a mass in her pelvis. Resection of this mass cured her bone disease. Looking at the wonderfully vital woman before me, I couldn't help but think of all the detractors of medicine who believe it a field that simply holds people together through their years of steady decline.

As my preceptor and her patient marveled about how long it used to take Mrs. Arnold (10 minutes they agreed) to move from the chair to the examining table, they spoke with an unmistakable pride in what they have faced together. So often in physicians' offices there seems to be a divide between doctor and patient. At the least there exists a divide concerning medical knowledge, which persists despite the downplay of physician paternalism in favor of patient autonomy. Perhaps it is that same divide that allows physicians to have a healing influence simply with their attention and presence. But there, in that room, I felt I was in the company of old friends. After we completed the necessary components of the physical exam, Mrs. Arnold asked my preceptor, "How's your granddaughter?" And then we moved on to the family pictures.

After the patient left my preceptor said, "Mrs. Arnold is one of the true success stories. It has been incredibly gratifying to be able to help her. I know it is hard not to focus on the drugs and diseases when you are in school. But that's why I am in medicine. This is what it is all about for me."

What has been very rewarding about doing outpatient medicine at this point in the year is that finally I have gained enough confidence to shift the focus from myself—the questions I need to ask, the skills I need to perform in the evaluation—and instead, to focus on the patient. I can reflect on what it means to be let into their rooms, into their lives. And I can see in the moment that what I say and do makes a difference.

I must admit it is refreshing to go back to the books. People have made this experience profound, and people have made it frustrating at times. The amazing thing is that when I review various disease states, my whole clinical year comes back to me. Primary pulmonary hypertension—Ms. C from Ob/GYN. Tuberous sclerosis—Ms. F from Medicine. Sagittal sinus thrombosis—Ms. H from Neurology. I confess I do not remember all their names. But if I picture on which side of the floor their rooms were located, or where their charts were kept, many of them do come back to me. And now my dispassionate texts are filled with their memory.

❤

# FEE

*Andrew Thomas*

A Connecticut cabinetmaker I used to work for once told me that the definition of a woodworker was a fellow who would talk longer and with more affection about his block plane than he would about his wife. Notwithstanding the comments of wives, this statement has less to do with the state of marriage than it does with the excellence inherent in a good block plane, for a block plane is a thing of grace. To the palm it feels like a handshake with a dear friend and to the eye its flowing lines recall an expensive Italian sports car. Like a good sonnet, each of a block plane's elements is in its perfect place—the whole could only be detracted from by any alteration. Better than a poem, which is the product of a single person, the design of the modern block plane is the fruit of centuries of modifications by hundreds of thousands of woodworkers, and in this tool, more than in any other, lies the soul of woodcraft.

Unfortunately, like most worthwhile things, a good hand plane is hard to come by. Declining production standards render most of the hand planes made today hardly worth the materials with which they are constructed. An outfit in Maine makes duplicates of the beautiful British and American tools that were made before World War II and charges a small fortune for them. Otherwise, the best way to come by a good plane is to haunt tag sales or, as it turns out, come to know Robert Smith.

Robert Smith was Wednesday afternoon's second appointment. As a third-year medical student halfway through the primary care rotation, my job was to get a history and examine him, determine what was wrong, and then present my findings to Dr. W, my preceptor.

Outside the exam room door I carefully read Mr. Smith's chart. I learned that he was a 73-year-old late-onset diabetic with six weeks of increasing fatigue and pain in the legs, the sort of nonspecific complaint that is common in a primary care setting. Mr. Smith rose to greet me. He was tall and straight with light blue eyes, pure white hair, and large capable hands. About him was the assurance most often seen in those who are capable and content with themselves. He introduced his wife, who turned out to be the local justice of the peace, and told me to call him Bob.

We chatted for a while and I learned that Bob was a cabinetmaker with a shop in New York City until 20 years ago when he moved his whole operation up to the small town where the clinic is located. As I've tried to build some furniture myself, we argued curly maple versus white oak and whether dowel joints are better than mitered ones until I looked at my watch, saw that the appointment was almost over, and asked what brought him to the doctor.

After that Bob's wife did most of the talking because, as she said, "Bob doesn't like to talk about what bothers him." What she said supported the vague complaints noted in the chart, Bob's physical exam was unremarkable so, somewhat puzzled, we ordered a panel of blood tests and a follow-up appointment was made for the following week.

Two days later the results of the blood tests arrived in the office. What we saw caused us to call Bob and change his appointment to an earlier day in the week. His creatinine levels indicated that his kidneys were going into failure and a measurement of the amount of oxygen- carrying-cells in his blood indicated mild anemia. Most alarming was the cause of the anemia; it didn't look like Bob was iron deficient or suffering from an internal bleed, but rather he was sequestering his iron in a protein called ferritin; this made the iron unavailable to the body to make red blood cells. The body will do this when it is fighting a severe infection, when it harbors a cancer or, as Dr. W noted, for unknown reasons.

When Bob came in early the next week I didn't have to review the chart; I knew it cold. He and his wife greeted me warmly. Since I wasn't sure how to convey all the things going on medically and Dr. W had his hands full with other patients, I allowed the interview to go slowly. I also must confess that I like to talk with old woodworkers. So Bob told me about his new shaping machine and railed about how expensive good tools were. I let on that I was looking for a block plane and asked if he had any tips on how to carve dovetail joints.

Later, when I asked him how he was and Mrs. Smith began to speak, he cut her off and gave me a clear concise history of how his symptoms had begun, progressed, and affected him over the past six weeks. I performed a focused physical exam that was entirely unilluminating and got Dr. W.

Dr. W came into the exam room, said hello, and set to explaining what the lab results meant in language similar to the language he had used to talk with me about them a couple of days before. The results of this would be predictable to anyone who has listened to his brother-in-law physicist explain quantum mechanics over Thanksgiving dinner. After 20 seconds, the Smiths' faces became blank, and when Dr. W finished up five minutes later and asked if they had any questions, they mumbled no.

One of the great advantages of being a third-year medical student is that only months before the same information that now confuses your patients confused you. I saw the Smiths' plight and retold them what the situation was. They understood me. They asked questions and when we were done Bob asked me if I'd like to swing by his shop after work. I said yes.

It is important to note that when I had asked Bob why he had come to see the doctor a big reason he gave was that it was interfering with his work in the shop. I took this with a grain of salt. At 73 I assumed that his son probably did most of the work and that he was more of a hobbyist. As he showed me around the shop, which was housed in a bright barn, I saw that I had been wrong. Bob was busier than most people half his age. On that day he was working on a series of display tables for a well-known store in Manhattan, while outside a truck full of custom furniture for individuals around the country was being loaded. His products were uniformly well made and beautiful.

After showing me the shop we talked about France, where Bob had been born, and the New York where he had spent most of his life. It became time to go and as we said good-bye Bob seemed to recall something; he went to a room in the back of the shop and returned with a Stanley block plane built in the 1920s. He told me I should have it and I accepted not knowing what to say.

As I drove home through the August twilight with the plane on the passenger seat beside my rumpled white coat, my thoughts swirled. So much was unknown about why this patient was ill and, then, there was no guarantee that when a diagnosis was made anything could be done. At the same time I was filled with the feeling that I had done something useful by finding the patient within the illness. And there to prove it, on the seat next to me, in the form of a hand plane, lay my first, unsolicited, fee.

# My Temple

*Jesse Selber*

I wake with a weird feeling in my gut. A remnant of dreams unremembered and a vague anxiety about past and future decisions. I get to the mirror and peer through the dusty reflection. He is not much different from the person I knew in college: not quite boy, not quite man, a little neater, a little more balanced. I tug at the skin of my cheek, "less creative, or just more obligated?" I wonder as I put myself together for the day.

My morning routine has slipped into ritual. I cinch the knot of my tie up to the neck, slide my beeper between the leather thongs of my suspenders, and pass the stethoscope gently over my head to rest on my shoulders.

I glance over at the self-portrait I began the night before, then to my guitar leaning up against the wall, and once more into the dusty mirror. The various compartments of my person bulge and recede in my own mind. I strain to align them, but soon resign to a cup of coffee and the peaceful veil of introspection that drapes the precious space between waking and work.

The drive to work: perhaps my finest hour. Never am I so completely myself as the hot coffee sloshes over my cold hands and the radio blasts something trying to be music. As I pull in to park, the final calibrations are made for my role as medical student: the proper degree of sanctimony, the edge taken out of my voice, the willingness to accept. I step into these vestments, not so much as a mask of surrender as a badge of honor, although depending on the day, it may be more the former.

The morning passes easily, mostly upper respiratory infections. The decisions are few; otitis or no, sinusitis or no, does suspicion warrant a strep test? I find interest in these mundane events in the interstices. I read the subtext and listen to words unspoken. Then there is the complicated patient. Columns of data and human emotions jump back and forth from foreground to background like school children vying for a teacher's attention. I do what I can with it all.

Finally the day draws to a close, the last patient waves goodbye and I sink back into my desk chair to finish a few notes. A contentment settles over me as I scan the desk for the previous patient's chart. My eyes land on a title in an open Newsweek—"World's Religions Espouse Quieting the Mind to Hear the Soul's Voice." I read on " . . . and in all these doctrines, separated by ice ages, languages and millennia, the inner voice urges followers to act with compassion."

I grin bitterly at how little I believe in the sorts of ideas for which people pray in churches and synagogues. In spite of this Godlessness, I do hear the voice of compassion. It asks me to touch patients gently, speak to them softly, and listen attentively.

Perhaps I know how to pray after all. And perhaps I have also found my temple.

# CHAPTER TWO

# LISTENING & TOUCHING

❤

*The manner of dealing with patients, of*
*winning their confidence, the art of listening to them . . . ,*
*of soothing and consoling them, . . .*
*—all this can not be learned from books.*

—Christian Albert Theodor Billroth
(*The Medical Sciences in the German Universities*, 1876)

Students acquire many essential skills as they evaluate patients in the office or clinic. Among the most important is to learn that patients benefit a great deal from empathetic listening, from a validation that their worries are important and deserve attention. They often need no more than to be heard. The treatment may be simple reassurance, which is often enough if it follows serious listening. The message cannot be an abrupt, "There's nothing wrong with you," but "I've heard your concern. I understand what you're worried about. I believe you will be all right." Patients often speak in metaphor, describing psychological and emotional pain in bodily terms. Listening to the patient's complaint with a poet's ear and knowing the patient's life situation, his work and home life, will reveal the meaning behind his words.

Students also learn the power of touch in conveying to the patient caring involvement. Be it sensitivity during a physical exam or simply a hand on the arm while taking a patient's history, direct touch can be therapeutic and healing in its own right.

# PAIN

*Margaret Talley*

You say it's your toe
It's changed and it hurts
Piercing as it strikes the front of your shoe
Once a crescent moon suspended
In soft translucent salmon sky
Now fractured, lifeless, opaque
You say it's your toe

She says it's your son
He's changed and it hurts
A growth, it sounds so promising
Born in his pancreas,
It snakes its way up, a choking vine
Strangling his clarity, his reason, all hope
She says it's your son

She says it's your grief
You've changed and it hurts
Anguish washes over you without warning
Like waves of nausea
Deep pain, dull like organ pain
A constant ache in your bones pain
You say it's your toe

❤

# A LITTLE EXTRA TIME

*Anonymous*

All it takes is a little extra time.

We're taught how to correlate stories and symptoms
with various diseases we've seen or read about,
then generate a differential diagnosis, including
all the zebras, only to immediately discard most
of them based on physical exam findings or lab
tests. Then we congratulate ourselves when we've
got *the* diagnosis, because it gives us something
we can treat. It's much more fulfilling to treat
an illness when you know its name.

Meanwhile, the patient becomes a secondary
consideration to the diagnosis. Of course, the
patient-diagnosis is actually one beast, but it's
easier to treat the diagnosis than the patient.

All it takes is a little extra time.

I'm young, I'm naïve, I'm still mostly idealistic.
I don't diagnose as efficiently as my seniors.
I don't know all of the treatments for all of the
diagnoses all of the time, or even some of the
treatments some of the time. That will come.
I have faith in the system. What I do have is
a view of the patient-diagnosis that is less
obstructed by the diagnosis. There really is a
patient in there if you dig beneath the surface
of the diagnosis. And all it takes to treat a
patient is a little extra time.

A little extra time to hold a hand, to console,
to give hope, to laugh, to listen. I haven't been

at this game very long, but I've learned that giving a little extra time can treat a patient for a minute, or a day, or a month. Maybe, over the years, the system will beat that out of me, but then again, I just might remember these early lessons. I will learn how to treat diagnoses, but for now, I'm learning how to begin to treat a patient. And all it takes is a little extra time

❤

## ANOTHER ANNUAL PE

*Amy Mastrangelo*

It's 2:30 on a Monday afternoon, the weekend is a distant memory by now. Oh great...another 50-something annual PE. Room 13—I grasp the chart, ahh...it's a thin one, that's a good sign...minimal pathology.

I open the door and say my lines, expecting to confirm the patient's willingness to be seen and examined by me before the real doctor comes in. The look of surprise, of fear, of crumbled hopes on his face startled me. I guess the nurse hadn't asked him if it would be okay if the med student interviewed him. Nevertheless he halfheartedly agreed, "Well, I guess it's okay, I'm just surprised." I reminded him of his rights—if he had an objection I would understand and the doctor would be happy to see him alone—after all, I could stand not to do another painstakingly tedious normal PE today. I was trying so hard not to get too defensive.

I started off with, "So we haven't seen you here since last year, any new problems?" Mr. Smith answered, "New problems, no." "Oh wonderful," I thought, "this is going to be like pulling teeth." So I asked the next logical question, "Any old problems?" Suddenly the patient's cold, hardened face softened. "Well . . . it's this insomnia, it's driving me crazy." I felt my muscles relax and found myself listening intently to his story—chronic insomnia for the past year. Sounds horrible, I remember a few, rare, restless nights and how frustrating and painful they can be, can't imagine how that would feel after months and months. He reviewed in detail his weekly schedule—works four 10-hour shifts per week, Sunday–Tuesday nights, Wednesday day. After work he invariably sleeps like a rock for the first five hours and then "pops up like a jack-in-the-box that has been wound up the whole night." Counting backwards, counting his breaths, listening to music or tapes of waterfalls, getting up, lying down, drinking warm milk, he's tried it all, nothing works, he just can't fall back to sleep.

He went on to articulately describe the repercussions of his lack of sleep—irritability, mood swings, lack of interest in his family, too much caffeine, "more alcohol than I probably should, about a 12-pack per week." Said he almost didn't come today because he felt so hopeless, but he just couldn't stand to think he'd feel this way the rest of his life. "Yikes," I thought "he just said the H word, hopeless." Had he thought about killing himself? Yes, just this past Saturday. He seemed relieved I asked. I reviewed the crisis services that were available. He was already familiar with them. He denied any active suicidal ideations and agreed to keep the list of phone numbers close by.

"So what's the cause of all this," I wondered. Almost in his next breath he volunteered that he "had never thought of himself as an anxious, stressed person, but . . . " then he began to rattle off his list of stressors: he's working on completing his bachelor's degree and is so close to finishing but feels absolutely overwhelmed, he has four grown children but lives with his girlfriend and her three teenagers, and work, oh work, he reviewed his new title and all the increased responsibility that goes along with it. I asked about depression (I thought it was blatantly obvious), he denied it. He had done a lot of reading and knew he met some of the criteria, but he felt his sleep problem was the cause of his troubles, not a symptom. He had been treated for depression two times before, only with counseling, no meds. He didn't feel further counseling would be helpful, he already knew "everything" they had to say. If only he could get some sleep, it would all be fine.

I reviewed the use of antidepressants as sleep aids, and then reflected on the signs and symptoms of anxiety and depression he described. I tactfully explained that I didn't feel medication alone would solve his problems. Although he couldn't bear to think of returning to counseling now, he surprisingly agreed it may be prudent in the future.

I transitioned into the physical exam, still trying to remain attentive to the problems at hand. Essentially normal PE, just like I expected; much more pathology than I had expected though.

After reporting my findings to the doctor, we went back in. He carefully assessed Mr. Smith's mental state; a trial of antidepressant for sleep and depression seemed warranted.

As I gathered together the mountain of paperwork, Mr. Smith pointed to my ID tag and said he had noticed that I went to school in Rochester. One of his sons goes to college there and he really seems to like it. He then smiled and thanked me, he felt like I was really listening to him. He was glad he had kept his appointment today. So was I.

# B.T.

*Cathryn McNamara*

My preceptor had warned me that she was a difficult patient and that I might not want to see her. But she was there, I was free, and he was seeing someone else. I thought, if nothing else, I could listen. I went to room 11, lifted her thick chart out of the plastic box and began to read. "A 47-year-old female with fibromyalgia, obesity, a history of depression, and lower extremity edema." Just seeing the word "fibromyalgia" caused my heart to race. The few patients I had seen with this condition had overwhelmed me. Having so many problems with so little relief caused them to be frustrated and dissatisfied with their care. Furthermore, they came seeking answers and cures, which I certainly did not have. I continued to read and when I had absorbed enough information about B.T., I closed the chart, prepared myself, knocked on the door, and entered the room. I was slightly surprised to find her sitting not on the exam table, but at the small desk usually occupied by the interviewer. She was a large, strong woman with red hair and a kind face. I introduced myself and asked her if she would be willing to see me before the doctor came in. She agreed and I pulled out the stool and sat across from her.

I asked her how she had been since her last visit. She answered forcefully. Her legs were still quite swollen and she was short of breath. She was extremely fatigued. Her narcotic prescription had been written for 50 tablets, not 100, and she'd need an additional script. She asked if we could please write it "D.A.W." as the brand she had been given by the pharmacy simply was not as effective. Initially, I was taken aback. She was obviously knowledgeable about her health, but that was not all. She made it clear that she was in charge. In addition, when I tried to ask her questions about her problems, she'd look at me almost in disbelief that I did not know the answers. The thought of cutting the interview short and calling on Dr. M for assistance did occur to me. I had, at times, done that if I sensed a patient was aggravated by talking with me. But, in this case, I decided to stay. I told her I would share the information with the doctor and asked her if she had any other concerns. A lot had happened since her last visit, she said. Most of it was related to issues for which she normally saw her ob/gyn. However, she thought we might like to keep up to date. I encouraged her to share the recent events and she began her story.

There had been a mix-up in communication about a screening test that led to a great deal of stress and worry. She went into great detail and finished by saying that furthermore, she had lost all confidence and trust in her doctors. "I don't believe anything anyone tells me anymore," she said.

As I listened to her tell this story, something quite remarkable happened. This woman whom I initially found to be closed, controlling, and almost overbearing had become a delicate, vulnerable, most human person more than willing to share her thoughts and fears with me. Whereas before she simply wanted to tell me what should be done, she now seemed to be looking to me for consolation. I empathized with her and apologized for the miscommunication. She told me that she had decided to see a surgeon as recommended. I encouraged her to do this. We spoke about a few other issues and I then left to discuss B.T. with my preceptor.

My preceptor sat patiently with me as I related the history and physical findings I had obtained. We then returned to the room together to complete the visit. When I entered this time, there was a different person sitting at the desk—not a stranger with an intimidating diagnosis ready to criticize me for my lack of knowledge, but a kind person with flaws and worries of her own. My preceptor addressed her concerns and again apologized for the miscommunication. Also, he did what he could to try to restore her faith in the medical professionals involved in her care. She then began telling him about the college courses she was taking over the telephone. Unfortunately she had had to drop one because of the stress and fatigue. She stated that she was going to keep working at it though, because it was important to her. In addition she mentioned that she had been slightly depressed recently and asked if she should go back on the antidepressant. She wondered if going back on the medication meant she was regressing. "It doesn't make me a bad person does it?" she asked. My preceptor assured her it was the right thing to do and that it did not in any way make her a bad person. He then concluded the visit and we walked out to the desk to write the prescription. As he was writing he said to me, "B.T. . . . her visits are a large part of her treatment." Without a doubt I knew what he meant. I then took her prescription down to the lab, where she was having blood drawn, and explained how she should take it. "Thank you," she said. "It was nice to meet you."

What B.T. wanted was someone to listen to her story. She needed to let her defenses down and relate her worries and fears, it seemed. Somehow that was therapeutic for her. Of course, I had heard time and time again that patients will often come to the doctor seeking an open ear and understanding. However, I never fully believed it. But, I thought, perhaps I had been wrong. And indeed, I have learned that B.T. is surely not alone. A little listening can go a long way.

# A GESTURE OF KINDNESS

*Andrew Brown*

I remembered driving to Cooperstown three weeks prior, Bob Marley blaring in my ears and thoughts of Doc Hollywood running through my head. Filled with expectations and happy to escape the confines of city life for a while. The leaves were still green and the air had just begun to take on the scent of winter that I love. Small towns and streams bright in the fall sunlight passing by my windows, fighting the urge to stop and take pictures of the barn animals.

"This is Andy Brown, a medical student working with me, would it be okay if he examined your mother?" I stood in her room silently standing behind and to the left of my preceptor. I stood there trying my best to absorb the interaction, to imprint the feelings and textures of the moment somewhere in my brain so I would not forget. Her daughter stood with her back to the window, fall foliage undulating brightly behind her through the window, and apprehensively smiled at us as we entered the room. She smiled because we were there to help her mother.

My preceptor greeted her and began to discuss issues surrounding the care of her mother. His demeanor instantly put her at ease. He was able to, in the space of 20 seconds, convey his support and understanding for her and her family. I had seen him do this countless times in the past weeks with patients of all ages. This remarkable quality that he and other physicians that I have been lucky enough to work with possess to convey and earn trust is always amazing to watch and be a part of. This time however his attentions were not focused on the patient, but on her family, because our patient was suffering from end–stage dementia.

The patient's pale blue eyes staring ahead in a look of perpetual surprise would occasionally focus on one of us and I could almost see recognition there. "I don't know," she said. Her daughter looked at us with tears in her eyes and told us how this tiny contracted woman had single-handedly saved her family and an entire barn full of animals from a fire 50 years previously, how she had raised her children and buried her husband, trying to communicate to us how she would like us to see her mother, how she still remembered her.

She and my preceptor stepped out of the room and I was left alone. I took a few moments to re-orient myself to my patient. Her shortly cropped gray hair was neatly combed back from her thin face. I remember wondering who in her family had taken the time to make her look so presentable. I began my exam and found myself trying desperately to connect with this patient. I wanted to know her as the person that was just described to me, to break down the wall her dementia had built up around her.

I began to examine her with the HEENT exam, progressing smoothly through the sequence that has become so familiar to me when, to my surprise, she commented that my hands were cold. I stopped my examination and apologized. Before I could continue she looked up into my eyes, smiled, and reached out for my hand. Before I could react she had gently grasped my right hand in hers and brought it to the crook of her neck to warm it. I remember standing there feeling slightly awkward at first but then wondering how many times she had done this for the members of her family, her children, her husband? Here I was a complete stranger and she was offering me this small gesture of kindness. She asked me why she was here and told me with tears in her eyes that she was ashamed of herself for not knowing. I told her she was in the hospital and would be going home the next day to be with her family. She let go of my hand and a single tear rolled down her face, "I don't know," she said and looked away.

I will be driving home tomorrow, Bob Marley still blaring in my ears, watching the leaves fall from the trees remembering the small moments that I was able to share with my patients, willing myself to never forget that small act, that instant of recognition that I was privileged to share.

# A RAY OF HOPE

*Nina Phatak*

A thinly clad leg moves
Exposing dusky feet and gnarled toes
Long ago encased in satin slippers
That lithely swayed to a lilting waltz
Wafting through a summer's eve

The stark sheet outlines skeleton legs
Lying in quiet repose
Once of glowing sinew and bunching muscle
 As they dashed after butterflies and rainbows
 Through daffodil fields

Tired eyes, in a withered, wrinkled face
Gaze at me
Reflecting memories of melting warmth
 Of solid proudness
 That beats in a mother's heart

Arms that fervently embraced a soldier
Hands once clasped against a shadowed jaw
Fingers that long ago soothed a child's tears
Now rest in mine
Heavily etched
Twisted bark

Weakly entwine
Subtle pressure speaks volumes of a bygone time
Yet silently whispers a current plea

Of twisting hope
Which begins with a passing touch
Silently bridging the chasm of despair

♥

# REVELATION

*Andrew Alexis*

As I reflect upon my primary care experience here at Bassett, I am reminded of the vast amounts I have learned in the short span of five weeks. While one of the most valuable things I have learned is how to manage such diverse patient concerns as, "I feel 'woozy' all over," and "Hey doc, am I ready for Viagra yet?," an even more important lesson comes to mind: the value of being an empathetic listener. In the midst of the many stresses and demands of a typical medical day, it is easy to underestimate the need to take time and listen. Failing to listen to a patient's concern, while trying to treat what appears to be clinically most significant is an easy trap to fall into. I found with time that simply offering my undivided attention and empathy would often help uncover the issues that really brought the patient into clinic, despite what was written on the triage note.

One example was a 42-year-old lady who came in to clinic complaining of fevers, cough, and sore throat for about two weeks. After a full workup that was for the most part unremarkable, I was ready to send her out with the unfulfilling diagnosis of "viral URI." It soon became clear that this cold of sorts wasn't the real reason she had come to visit the doctor. Looking unsatisfied with my decision not to treat her illness, she proceeded to volunteer that her "coming down with something" is probably related to all the stress she's been under lately. Feeling somewhat annoyed by the fact that I was behind with two patients waiting, I sat down to listen to her story, albeit reluctantly. She began to tell me about how her publishing business had fallen into dire straits, while relations with her husband had become increasingly strained in the past few months. As I sat quietly, nodding my head and looking into her eyes, her thoughts and emotions became more forthcoming, and she began to cry. Feeling useless, I offered her the only comfort I could—handing her a tissue and lending my ear to listen some more. It was then that our one-sided conversation turned to the issue that concerned her most. With tears flowing, she described how she had been feeling depressed for months and had lost all interest and energy for the things that she loved. She felt personally responsible for the demise of her business and her troubled marriage. She admitted feeling inadequate with respect to her role as a wife and mother of two children. On several occasions, she even contemplated ending what she felt was a worthless life. Not prepared for such a revelation, I sat silently for what felt like an awkward eternity, before assuring her that her life is indeed worth living.

After a pause, she replied, "You really think so?"

"Yes. I know so," I responded, reaching for her hand.

As she squeezed my hand tightly the rush of tears began to gradually subside, and she dried her watery eyes. Then, mustering up a smile, she said,

"Thank you," in a soft and vulnerable voice.

"Thank you?" I thought to myself.—"For what? I didn't do anything."

It was then that I realized that my seemingly useless contribution to our interaction, may actually have been as beneficial as the antidepressant I would eventually prescribe her. The simple reassurance that someone was willing to listen to her concerns and sympathize with her was in itself a therapeutic measure; an opportunity to help that would have easily been lost had I failed to recognize her need to be heard.

From this experience, I am reminded of the power and importance of listening. As one of the most valuable skills that can be employed by a physician, it is easily overlooked or underestimated. As this encounter proved, simply listening with a patient and empathetic ear can help reveal substantial concerns that would otherwise be missed. Experiences such as this one underscore the diverse roles we as physicians are intended to play—including that of healer, counselor, teacher, and friend.

♥

## THE UNSPOKEN

*Fenny Lin*

The face of the person perched on the examining table looked familiar, but I could not remember when I had last seen those intelligent, sharp, eyes. Mrs. Plummer explained that we had met a week ago when she had accompanied her 95-year-old mother to the clinic. Now she herself was here for a visit to follow her diabetes. After reviewing her glucose control, I asked Mrs. Plummer if she had any other concerns. In a very matter-of-fact manner, she began to talk about her mother. As she described the problems she was facing, I started to remember the previous week's meeting.

That day, I had met a petite, serene-looking, woman with a mild demeanor and soft smile, accompanied by her 71-year-old daughter. Mrs. Plummer had acted as her mother's voice since Mrs. Smith was going deaf and needed new hearing aids. Mrs. Smith had several items on her agenda, which her daughter brought to my attention. But the most striking moment of that visit came at the end of our talk, right before I left the room. In a lowered tone, Mrs. Plummer asked for the doctor's and medical student's help in persuading her mother not to attend a granddaughter's wedding out West, explaining that the trip was too long and that she did not think her mother could handle the long drive because "even the trip to the doctor's office makes my mother exhausted."

My inexperience and reflexive trust in Mrs. Plummer's understanding of her mother's condition led me to advocate her position when I spoke to my attending. Her concern seemed well grounded and reasonable; she was afraid that the trip would exacerbate her mother's frail health. My attending, however, had a different perspective. He said, "Go to the wedding! It'll make her happy. At her age, what's the worst that can happen? She might die on the road, instead of at home." Even before he finished speaking, I realized how right he was. We can worry so much about patients dying that we forget that living involves much more than keeping the blood circulating. The human spirit, if depressed, can be far more difficult to correct than, say, a low hematocrit. Time and again, in the past few weeks, I have seen that patients with similar medical conditions may make different decisions about their treatment. The best medical fix may not necessarily be the best solution for a particular patient's problem. My impression of Mrs. Plummer shifted slightly. Although I understood her genuine concern, I suspected a small element of unconscious selfishness in her desire to leave her mother at home for convenience. But the doctor did not give Mrs. Plummer a medical excuse to dissuade her mother from going to the wedding.

Now, a week later, I was hearing the other side of the story that had been unspoken at the last visit. Mrs. Plummer explained that her mother was deteriorating rapidly in her ability for self-care. Most worrisome of all was that she was mixing up her medications. Mrs. Smith adamantly refused her daughter's suggestion that she move into her house, seeing that as a symbol of dependency and helplessness. Already, Mrs. Plummer and her husband check up on her mother three times a day, but even these measures seemed inadequate. "When I'm not at her house," she explained, "I'm still constantly worrying about her. Plus, my daughter is medically unstable, so I am always taking either my mother or my daughter to the hospital." With none of Mrs. Plummer's siblings helping to take care of their mother, she was angry, frustrated, worried, and felt helpless, depriving her of restful sleep at night. During our conversation, she had been very composed. But when I hesitated before leaving the room, Mrs. Plummer cracked and the emotions behind her story finally tumbled out. Again, her calm demeanor had fooled me. She had spoken about her feelings, but she had not yet had that cathartic release that came with simply crying. Mrs. Plummer refused an antidepressant to help her deal with the pressures, but talking about her distress had clearly been therapeutic. I am a good listener, but I was quickly learning that hearing the unspoken, the suggested, was just as important as registering a patient's actual words.

These two encounters made me question the idea of patient advocacy. Being a patient advocate seems an easy task, but that ideal is complicated when the doctor must support two patients' wishes that are in direct conflict with one another. While Mrs. Smith clearly should not miss her granddaughter's wedding, we also cannot ignore Mrs. Plummer's emotional well-being. In the long run, will Mrs. Smith accept a 24-hour home health aide or will she see that as compromising her independence as well? Even though no clear answers present themselves, knowing the whole story is far more helpful than having only a simplistic, one-sided, perspective. Often, obtaining the whole story requires learning to hear the unspoken messages.

CHAPTER THREE

# PATIENTS

♥

*Clearly no disease can exist without*
*a person to suffer from it. A disease is an abstraction.*
*The patient is the concrete reality.*

—A. E. Clark-Kennedy
(Kelly M, *Archives of Internal Medicine*, 1962)

The privilege of knowing intimately the body and soul of patients, of being entrusted with their innermost fears and worries as well as having access to their physical being, is unique to medicine. Physicians learn the art of maintaining enough distance from their patients so as not to become personally overwhelmed by their troubles and, hence, lose objectivity and perspective. Yet, the effective physician learns to get close enough to understand patients' feelings and experiences. Such empathetic attentiveness is the essence of the art of medicine.

Although some patients initially express disappointment at being asked to see a student, they almost always find these same neophyte physicians to be supportive listeners. The students have the luxury of time and, perhaps out of a sense of inadequacy, are more inclined to "just listen" while patients talk. Out of such experiences come remarkable stories by students showing their appreciation of the people they encounter.

.

# I Want to See the Doctor

*Erica Shoemaker*

"No, I want to see the doctor."

"You see, I've brought this whole list of questions and I want to talk to the doctor. I want to ask her about my vitamin pills. Is it all right to dissolve them in water because they are so hard for me to swallow. And my arthritis . . . "

"Well, if you insist . . . if there is no way around it. Then I suppose you will have to do."

"You go ask her how I can lose weight. I'm losing my figure, you see, and I wonder if it might have something to do with the ice cream."

"Well, I eat the whole container, I'm afraid. It's just that it's there in my freezer and it's so hard to stop. I didn't used to look like this, but how would you know? It's true though, I was lithe and light on my feet. When I was a young lady, I lived in Greenwich Village and danced with Ruth Saint-Denis, although I doubt you know who that is, but in my day she was really quite the latest thing, you see. We gave concerts in the park and did gypsy dances and Oriental dances, especially the Turkish dance which was my favorite because you wore swishy purple skirts and red brassieres and I was really quite good, you see. It didn't last long because I was so good that Madame Saint-Denis she got jealous and I had to leave, so I went back home with my mother and we visited the grave of my brother killed in the Great War. A pilot, a brave pilot, but the Germans shot him down and he came back to us nothing but a body. We had a full service for him in the Presbyterian Church with an oak casket and white lilies and yellow roses and . . . nobody grows lilies anymore why is that?"

"Where was I . . . I can't remember. Why is it I can't remember anything? Ask the doctor why I can't . . . hold anything in my head . . . or remember? Where is my list?"

"Breathe. I can't breathe easily now. You see, it's blocked up like that. Pfft. The doctor tells me it's because of my cigarettes. I sneak them on the back porch, but I want to ask her about the cod liver oil because when I was taking that cod liver oil I never got pneumonia. I think the world of cod liver oil, don't you? When I was a girl, my mother used to make us drink three tablespoons of cod liver oil each night before bed, and I don't understand why she told me not to take the cod liver oil like I used to do when I was a girl and my mother was going to be a doctor just like you, you see, but then she met my father. She said he was the handsomest man she had ever seen and he used to sing to her outside her window and it made my grandfather so mad she had to marry Papa just to shut him up. Mama died and Papa had to run the whole farm himself, we had cattle and hogs and we grew corn and hay for feed and Papa would take us out into the field and hold us by our arms and whip us around and around we got so dizzy, but it was fun, more fun than any Ruth Saint-Denis whirligig dance anyway somehow."

"The list . . . where is my list? I can't find it, but I want to tell that doctor how mad I was when she told me to move into a home. I get along just fine, you see, I have friends around the corner who help me shop and who cares if I can't get up and down the stairs so good. I'd like to see her climb my stairs—it's 24 stairs total, with two landings and I can make it just fine if I take a couple of breaks and pet Millie for a few minutes. I showed her I could manage because I didn't come in for a few years after she said that. I'd like to see her when she's 92; can you believe that—92 years old and only one greatgrandson. He's a genius and handsome he has nice teeth, like you and he's going into the pilot's Air Force school and I want to see him graduate and fly those planes around and around like whirling dervishes."

"You go tell the doctor I want to live another four years."

"Tell her to make me live another four years."

💜

# L.J.

*Clinton Wright*

Pleasant-looking,
Young woman.
Twenty-nine.
Pale skin, hair
Long and brown.
Tattoos, poorly made.
Like a child had doodled
When she wasn't looking.
When she was too stoned to care.

Running away.
No more beatings.
No more cheatings.
Bye-bye abuse. Left it in the mid-west,
With the strip malls and the Ponderosas
Old car parts in the living room
Smell of whiskey and cat pee.
A cold hand across the face.

Barmaid with four children (left one in Cleveland)
Always had been
In the bar, real people,
Or people being real. Forgot which.
Now a new start.
On the road to wellness.
No more drinking, no more nasty stuff.
Still working in a bar. Can't change your whole self.
Not that fast, anyway.

H-O-P-E spelled out across her knuckles.

Hadn't helped.

Hope springs eternal.

♥

## OVERDOSE

*Kristel Kalissaar Hunt*

It's 12 o'clock midnight. The phone rings—once, twice, three times. It starts to get real annoying. Then it hits me; the phone's ringing! I weightlift the receiver slowly to my ear.

As expected, no personal calls at this hour—it's the ER all right. A kid with a caffeine overdose, not a suicide attempt, just wanted to get high—a high school kid, I believe. Ann, the R.P.A. on call tonight, already checked with Poison Control and apparently caffeine overdose requires 10–12 hours of close monitoring, as there is a great chance of delayed tachycardia. Which means he needs to be admitted. Two nerves, one synapse: there's only one empty ICU bed left, and no space at all on the floor—unless someone died. Just great.

"So you mind checking this scumbag out, Kristel?" He sounds pretty groggy. Needs his beauty sleep, I guess. I try to sound enthusiastic in my response. "And remember to wear your gloves." He's grinning. I can hear it. "Call if you have any questions, OK?" OK.

I wrap my pet snake around my neck, try to steal a quick glimpse at the overdose section of the "Primary Care Secrets" to see if anything else besides chugging lots of charcoal is absolutely mandatory to treat a caffeine overdose, find my clogs (one under the bed, the other finally located between the paws of our yellow lab and suspiciously moist) and am on my way out. It had been raining elephants and giraffes all night, and had finally stopped; the golden sliver of a moon was almost penetrating the clouds. Lungs expanding, I start the car.

. . .

To tell you the truth, I was surprised when I first saw the culprit who had driven me out of bed and into the dark night. I had expected a good-looking, pony-tailed and body-pierced smart-butt guy, loud and obnoxious and uncooperative. The kind where you just have to set some chord vibrating in them or else they won't even open half an ear. But here . . . I had one scrawny little guy, with half-an-inch thick glasses and pretty bad acne. Hmmm . . . pretty far off, I guess.

We started talking. I liked him immediately, almost instinctively—kind of the way you would like a puppy that's smaller and weaker than the others and has a really tough time getting its share of food. Bill had been pushed around in his life a fair bit as well, definitely more than his fair share. His father, one of the all-time favorite polysubstance abusers in jail for credit card fraud, his mom somewhere in the Southwest and very much out of the picture, he had been in foster care for the last five years. In this one family for the last two. And his relationship with his foster parents had been far from good from early on—and beyond the teenage rebellion stuff. Bill suspects that they had taken him in for the extra money—not unlikely, I suppose. And then the ex-straight A student starts drinking and smoking pot on weekends, his drinking buddies his only friends at school, starts skipping classes to get high in the nearby parking lot and failing most of his classes. He never tries any of the hard stuff, but drinks most days now, just beer, but weekends as well as weekdays. His tolerance level is still pretty low, so it doesn't take him more than four beers to get sick to his stomach—at which point he usually stops. Recently he's taken up caffeine pills, guarantees an "easy fix"—a good high that comes relatively cheap. At least he can afford it from his allowance without resorting to alternative methods of making money, whatever they may be.

He throws up, misses the urinal that he had sitting on his lap. I go and steal him a pair of scrubs and there's a shadow of a smile on his face.

No friends. No family—his one brother who he grew up with god-knows-where. Sucks in sports. Likes computers, but the one in school is not accessible after-hours and he sure can't afford one. Nothing to do. No one to talk to. Would it be normal NOT to satisfy the five of nine (DSM-IV) here? I'm not sure. And so I sit by his bed, watch him sip on the charcoal and listen to his story. Keep wondering if anyone had really heard it before. The "scumbag" has long since drifted away, and I'm left sitting with a sad and lonely child. It's raining again.

♥

## GROUND RULES

*John Harrison*
*(with assistance by an anonymous elderly lady)*

I don't want a pelvic.
You won't check my stools.
You can't touch my breasts.
Because those are the rules.

My back is so sore
and my hearing is gone.
My eyesight is fading
and I haven't got long.

My children have grown
and my husband is dead.

Silence surrounds me
alone in our bed.

Were I twenty years younger
I might have complied.
Now I'm too old to worry
yet too young to die.

## Medicating Life?

*Aimee Vafaie*

He showed me his wife's picture. I'm not sure how it came up, really. I had just met Mr. Johnson, this sweet elderly carpenter, and we were making small talk, and laughing at each other's jokes, when he mentioned her. She died just a few months ago, in her sleep. She was beautiful and smart and talented and charming and delightful. In the black-and-white picture he has clearly carried for decades, she is young and angelic, with a smile that is lighting up her young husband's face. He confided in me that he misses her. His blue eyes sparkled with delight . . . and unshed tears.

In the next room was another sweet elderly man, a dairy farmer, whose wife was dying from Alzheimer's disease. The doctors in the clinic often lovingly describe their favorite patients as "the salt of the earth"—Mr. Carney was just such a man, and he was holding on to every bit of responsibility to his wife that he could. It had been a struggle to convince him to place her in a nursing home, to leave his beloved in the care of a stranger. With pain on his face, he told me about her deterioration. She had lost her memory, her control of her bowels and bladder, and now was having difficulty eating. He feels sure that she cannot eat unless he feeds her, so he travels 15 miles to her nursing home three times a day to spoon-feed her mush, and he rarely goes anywhere else. She only sometimes recognizes him, as he lovingly tends to her. He can't reach her. He watches in anguish as she loses everything she was. He will never have a memory of their happiness together that is not tainted by this decay.

As he talked, the room became darker, and the air heavier. Tears filled my eyes, as I struggled to look professional. But his eyes were dry and his face unchanged. He is helpless, his life is shrouded in darkness and heavy with the slow death of his wife. We tried to proceed to his health, which was why he was here, after all. There was unspoken guilt on his face, for he is still healthy and strong, while she falls apart. It was time to send him for another colonoscopy, and he chuckled dryly at the mention of cancer screening. "It doesn't matter once Ann is gone," he shrugged.

Of course we could call this depression. We could talk about his feelings in clinical terms and say he was still functioning, though retreating from society. His affect was blunted, and he is unable to detach sufficiently from his wife's disease. And we could offer medication to help him cope. I have always believed that life is what you make of it, and that happiness can be found, often in bringing joy to others, but seeing this man and feeling his weight, I felt hopeless, too. He needed something I felt completely unable to find or offer. How could I, a young woman, newly married, and with a life full of hope and dreams for future happiness, tell this man whose happiness seems all behind him . . . how could I tell him anything? I was suddenly so terrified of being in his place someday, with nothing to hold on to or look forward to, and with everything I had build my life and happiness around, seemingly gone forever.

Like Mr. Carney I clearly have much to learn about accepting my own powerlessness and coming to terms with loss. I couldn't easily find a happy ending to this story. Once his wife has passed away, we hope Mr. Carney will be able to finally relinquish this pain and responsibility, and find purpose and happiness again. He has children and grandchildren who love him dearly. He is healthy and strong, kind-hearted, and hard-working. He has always been a stubborn fighter. As his physicians we actually can foster these strengths. For now, we can offer support and advice and maybe some medication. And we will keep a close eye on him and help him make this transition. We can be his friends, and learn from each other, and hope it is enough.

## The Other Side of the Diagnosis

*C. P. Krishnamurthy*

I'm up again. Its 4:30 and the last time before that was 2:30 and the time before that 2:20. You'd think that after the past week I'd be able to sleep for a day but I just can't. My husband on the other hand is asleep. That's no surprise. He hasn't made it through the 10 o'clock news in years. If he didn't get so cranky I think I'd wake him up, but the last thing I need is for him to be upset with me. I'll just get up and get my day going early. As I'm pulling myself out of bed my hands reach for my stomach as a force of habit. It still hurts. I won't be able to cancel that doctor's appointment. This'll be my third visit in less than a week.

Two weeks ago I fell while working in the garden and I thought I hurt my shoulder. Three days later I felt this pain in my back. It didn't bother me during the day but when I lay down it started again. I told my husband about it and he thought it might be my kidney. So I went into the clinic the next day and saw that new lady. She's a nurse-practitioner and she never interrupts me when I'm talking, the way those doctors do, so I like her. I always get so flustered when they rush me and I forget what I want to say. When I remember I get all upset and worry for days. She told me that my back must have gotten hurt a little bit when I fell and that I should just take a pain pill or two with dinner. Then I remembered that I had gotten this funny pain in the belly the night before and I told her. And that when I had to go to the bathroom not very much came out. Well, she just told me to keep using that powder and use a laxative when I needed to.

A day or two later that pain in my belly felt much worse. It's right below my ribs, and I usually only felt it when I was lying down. It's a burning pain, and I started rubbing it to make it feel better. The next morning I woke up and it still hurt and I hadn't gone to the bathroom in almost two days, so I called the clinic to try to make an appointment. I decided that this time I would see a doctor. I wrote down what I wanted to say, so I wouldn't forget it no matter how much he rushed me. I got to the office, waited my turn, and then sat in the room thinking about all the bad things that I could have. When the door finally opened, it wasn't the doctor. It was some medical student. He asked me some questions and I tried to answer him. I don't even know if I told him everything—I was just so worried about what the doctor was going to tell me. He did a quick examination on me and left, telling me that the doctor would be by in a couple minutes. By the time he finally came back with the doctor, my hands were continually rubbing my belly and I knew it must be bad, whatever I had. The doctor asked me a few questions about my stomach. He had the student check my stool for occult blood and I didn't know what that meant until he told me to roll on my side. It was uncomfortable but so was having to go home and try to sleep through all of his. Then the doctor said, "So you've been having this pain in your stomach but it doesn't hurt all the time, usually only when you're lying down. And you think you might have a problem with your kidney because your back hurt?" He flipped through my chart. "And you have a history of episodes of stomach pain. You've also had periods of depression and anxiety." Then he gave the medical student a look and I could swear the two of them smirked, like they didn't believe that it really hurts. He started asking me all these questions about other things. Do I live by myself, am I lonely, do I worry a lot, does anyone that I am close to work in the health profession. All these questions got me more nervous than the interrupting ever did. I don't remember a thing that anyone said. They left the room and came back in a minute. The doctor told me that I was in fine health, that my back pain was probably because of my fall, and to keep on taking the pain pill when my back hurt. How could I be in fine health and feel like this, I wanted to say. But all I actually said was, what about my stomach? He told me that all their findings were negative, but if it would make me feel better they could draw some blood and run some tests, and I would be called if anything was wrong. They took their blood, ran their tests, and some secretary called me three days later and told me that everything was normal.

Everything couldn't have been normal, but I decided I was going to live with this. I'd tough it out, the pain would go away, and I'd be fine. I wasn't going to need any doctor and I wasn't going to go back to the office. But then I spoke to Janice down the street, the one who lives up here in the summer and in Florida the rest of the year, and she was telling me about her friend Susan whose stomach hurt and had to spend a week in the hospital. So I got nervous and worried for two days until yesterday, when my husband forced me to call the doctor. And I did, and I made an appointment. For this morning. Which is why I can't sleep, because I'm nervous, not about my health or this very real pain in my stomach, but about being told that everything is normal.

# Epiphany

*Elizabeth Gerstner*

SORE THROAT

That's what the phone slip said.

"OK," she thought. "I can do sore throat. It is either viral or bacterial and most likely viral. Simple."

Having seen numerous sore throats before, she would be able to do a really good history and physical, including all the pertinent positives and negatives, and impress her preceptor. Most important, she would be able to offer suggestions for a course of action—that seemed to be the most impressive feat for a medical student. With most of the patients who came to the clinic she felt confused or completely at a loss as to what to do with them although she didn't let on that she was confused, of course. Other times nothing seemed to be done and yet the patient was told to return in 2–3 months. What was the point of having the patient return so often if you were not going to do anything for him? She found it incredibly frustrating and was glad she was young and healthy and didn't have to go see a doctor herself.

She briefly skimmed through the thin chart hanging on the door of "sore throat." It contained the brief story of a 31-year-old woman without any serious medical problems other than she apparently had had numerous sore throats in the past. She knocked briskly on the door, eager to get started on her successful operation.

"Come in."

She walked into the room with her most congenial and sympathetic smile programmed onto her face.

"Hello, I am a medical student working with the doctor today. Do you mind if I speak to you first while the doctor is busy with another patient?" she inquired brightly while sitting down without waiting for an answer.

"Will this take longer? No, I'd rather just see the doctor."

"Oh, he might be several minutes, though," she stammered confusedly. A patient saying no to her? She was here to learn from these patients and how was she supposed to learn and impress her preceptor if patients said no?

"No, I just want to see the doctor," came the reply and the woman turned away to stare at the wall.

She quickly got up and left the room, muttering "Well, I hope you feel better" on her way out. There! That'll show her! How triumphant to take the high road and show the patient she was not bothered by being turned away. She had plenty of other patients more worthy of her attention anyway. A simple sore throat was really a waste of valuable leaning time anyway. She thought back over the patients she had seen in the past couple of days, reminding herself of all the interesting cases she had helped. However, similar to sore throat lady, very few of them, if any, had seemed to appreciate her.

There was the 30-something guy with hypertriglyceridemia and hyperlipidemia whose entire diet consisted of only hamburgers—except for breakfast. For breakfast he would eat a poptart with cinnamon—not with fruit filling because that would probably remind him of actually eating something healthy. She had asked him if he considered expanding his diet to include some vegetables and he had said, "No, why should I? I am very healthy other than this high cholesterol and that seems to be controlled by that medication I am taking. And besides, sometimes I have lettuce and tomato on my burger so I do get some veggies." It was hopeless. He was not going to change his habits until he had an MI she thought bitterly.

OK, she continued to herself, there was that one guy I made a connection with. But that, too, had not panned out. He had turned out to be psycho. Well, of course that wasn't really the most PC way to put it but it was basically true. He had appeared to be an easygoing, healthy, athletic guy in for a regular checkup, and the interview had started off really well or so she thought. They had been chatting and he was opening up to her, telling her how he had just turned 51 and was feeling old. In her mind she labeled him as mid-life crisis and sat patiently listening to him rattle on about his life like she thought she was supposed to. Every so often her mind would wander—would she go swimming or play squash at the gym tonight? When she returned, he would be looking at her expectantly, so she smiled and nodded and he would launch into another round of somatic complaints. Everything seemed to bother him from his knees to his stomach to his head. He wanted to be checked for diabetes, high cholesterol, heart disease—everything the evening news made patients scared to death of. She slowly realized that his rather stoic appearance was deceiving and she quickly grew tired of his complaining. He kept asking her questions about growing old and what limits his health might place on his day-to-day activities. How was she to know? She was only 25 and had no clue what it was like to be 51! What did he expect from her? She couldn't answer his innumerable questions! She finally managed to extract herself from the room and find her preceptor. She also began worrying what he might say since she had spent so much time with the patient. These doctors were on a tight schedule and could not afford to have some lowly med student tripping up their precisely timed routine. All in all, it had been a frustrating experience and not an effective use of her time, especially when she heard she had missed seeing a case of pityriasis rosea since she had wasted so much time with psycho-patient.

She gave herself a shake to clear her mind of these unpleasant thoughts. So what if the patients didn't seem to pay any attention to her or listen to her suggestions? She was trying her best to help them and if they didn't want to hear it was their loss! She gave herself another shake and picked up the chart for the next patient.

He was a 76-year-old man with CHF whose EF was 15%. Wow, I've never seen anyone outside the hospital with an EF as low as 15%, she thought. She brushed past the wheelchair parked outside, knocked on the door, and went in. He was sitting on the exam table looking surprisingly undistressed. Although he did appear frail, he seemed cheerful and eager to see a new young face. He reminded her of her own grandfather. His plump, round wife was sitting on the chair at his side with his eight plus medications laid out neatly in her lap. She gave them her cute smile she used for elderly patients to appeal to their "grandparental" side and, after introducing herself, opened the interview with the usual open-ended questions she had been taught.

"How are you feeling today?"

"Oh fine, doctor," it gave her a little thrill to hear patients call her doctor even though she righteously assured herself she had introduced herself as a student and not an M.D. yet. "I just can't get around like I used to."

This last statement let her launch into her automated "CHF question-line." What limited him (pain or trouble breathing?), what activities made him short of breath, how many pillows did he sleep with, etc. She knew this down pat from having seen so many cases on the inpatient service. She was surprised to learn that even just getting out of bed or shaving caused him significant distress. It was hard to believe since he looked so well just sitting there talking to her. Sure his breathing became a little labored when he spoke excitedly about something but he still reminded her of her grandfather who was a very spry 86. He was especially agitated when he talked about seeing his twin granddaughters graduate from Colgate in June.

"How am I going to make it there if I can barely get out of bed to shave, doc?" he protested. "You've gotta do something for me!" His blue eyes stared at her with an intensity and desperation she had not seen before and did not know how to respond to. She was momentarily speechless in the face of this man's vehement need to have somebody help him. His wife started chiming in about her husband's limitations and their desire to do anything possible to help him get better.

"You gotta make me better, doc! I used to bike and swim laps around these young folk. You gotta make me better!" he repeated vigorously. She stared at this raw emotion with little ability to defend herself. She realized she knew nothing about this man or why he was even in heart failure. She had not even bothered to delve further into his history than the last entry in the chart. She felt incredibly young and inadequate, a feeling she hated, so she took the practical approach and decided to go over his medications with him. It would bring the discussion down to a more concrete topic and avoid her having to keep looking into his hungry eyes (she could look at the labels on his medicine bottles). It turned out he was taking almost every possible medication to improve the function of his heart. He was not taking a beta blocker, though, and her spirits rose. She could now suggest he try a beta blocker. It would impress her preceptor and maybe even make him feel better.

"Well, there is one more medication you could try," she said triumphantly.

"It's not that one that slows your heart is it?" he asked. "I tried that one and my lungs filled with water."

Against her will, her face fell. There was not much else to offer this man. He was not going to recover. She didn't even know if he would be healthy enough (alive even?) to see his granddaughters graduate. Her eyes darted around the room trying to avoid his searching, desperate gaze. She muttered something about getting the doctor to come in now and slunk out of the room, tripping over her stool and banging her elbow on the exam table as she exited. Once outside, she realized she hadn't even examined him.

# REFLECTION ON AGED PATIENTS

*Christina Treece*

On my fourth day at the clinic, I met Catherine Cardoza, a 101-year-old woman, and the oldest person I have ever met. I have had a fascination with elderly people since I began seeing them more this year as a medical student on the wards. Never having spent time with my grandparents (who all died before I was born—or lived on the other side of the world), some part of my life has been neglected, and the need has been met this year. Others had warned me against the old "gomey" patients—"they smell funny, stick to pediatrics." But in a way, I feel that elderly patients (meaning 80 years or older) are more rewarding and endearing than even the sweetest babies and toddlers. In some ways they can be childlike in their innocence and simplicity, as Mrs. Cardoza ("dear lady") was—she weighed about 75 pounds, could only remember our conversation for about 30 seconds, and then repeatedly asked the same questions in a high-pitched squeaky voice. Her granddaughter and caretaker had brought her into the clinic because she had had a cellulitis on her forearm and now had several bruises. They doted on her, smiling and laughing, and we all continually reassured her that the bruises she looked at in surprise every minute or so on her arm were okay. "What's that?" she'd say pointing to her elbow, "did I do something wrong?" until finally we helped her pull her sweater back over the troublesome arm, and she could forget to be upset about the ugly marks.

Mrs. Cardoza and some of the other patients I've seen are so completely responsive to attention and warmth. Most children (unless they've been in a hostile environment) will be carefree and self-absorbed, oblivious to the silly smiles and attention I give them; they are serene in being the center of the universe. With the older patients, I am gratified with the feeling that my role as a medical student is an important one, and that the patients readily accept what I am able to give them—simply time, respect, and a willingness to listen to their stories.

That sweet innocence coming out of Mrs. Cardoza's eyes was not that of an untouched simpleton. She had seen the world, lived a life, since 1899 in fact! She had emigrated from Italy in the early part of the century, and spent the rest of her life in upstate New York, raising a large family through the Depression, and ultimately inspiring great love and devotion in her family and those taking care of her.

She died one week after I saw her, in her sleep I heard, her spirit flitting away from her frail body. All the nurses and doctors in the clinic smiled and stopped to remember her when we heard the news; there was no sadness in such a peaceful passing away of a long and well-lived life.

Another older patient who I met at the clinic was a different character altogether. Mr. Masters had atrial fibrillation and poorly controlled diabetes, and he had had a small stroke about one year ago. He had decided recently to stop taking his coumadin, as he felt that it made his legs swell. Nurses and doctors had cajoled him and threatened him, but he had decided to take three aspirin per day instead. On the day that he was in the clinic for routine follow-up, I was supposed to initiate the history and physical. I had been running a little late, so I entered his room to be greeted with him yelling: "I don't wait for anyone, I won't wait for the Pope." He announced that he fired all doctors that made him wait more than 10 minutes. He proceeded to tell me that he had nearly fallen on the walk in from the parking lot, but a security guard had caught him. Mr. Masters was nearly deaf, so we yelled back and forth for a while. He was infuriatingly stubborn and refused to consider all my proposals—that he use a cane, reconsider coumadin as he might have another stroke, or see the eye doctor. I pulled his socks off to examine for pedal edema and saw that two toes were already gone, and the others were inflamed and oozing. This was not all damage from diabetes—he told me how the two toes had been shot off during World War II. He also told me that he had worked as a bookbinder for years on Fifth Avenue in New York and that he used to have a lot of clout. He regretted that he no longer had clout but said that he was still going to decide what was best and when it was to be done. Part of me wanted to argue with him and make him take the antibiotics that he refused for his infection. But still, I had to respect his determination and independence. His mind was as sharp as ever, and he simply refused to acknowledge the indignities of his body. He told me that he had to die from something and that he would decide for himself what treatments were acceptable.

Mr. Masters who had been so crotchety and unreasonable, thanked me on his way out and said not to pay attention to all the nonsense he talked because I was going to be very good one day. I felt grateful and a little sad as I watched him slowly leave. But there was nothing to pity, and I had nothing but respect for this "difficult" patient who could teach me so much about dignity and inner strength.

CHAPTER FOUR

# Caring & House Calls

♥

*He is the best physician who is the best inspirer of hope.*

—Samuel Taylor Coleridge (*Table Talk*, 1831)

Encounters with patients as they cope with serious illness are powerful learning experiences. The opportunity to witness the devotion of long-time partners to the support of an ill spouse can be even more inspiring. Students learn that caring is always possible and necessary even when cure is unattainable.

In the Bassett primary care clerkship the teacher often invites the student along on visits to attend patients in nursing facilities, the local jail, or the patient's own home. The home visit provides important insight into the patient's capacity for self-care and the status of his support systems. It also brings the caregiver into the patient's world—a gesture that, as patients will note, has great meaning. The students thereby learn to appreciate the value of continuity of care and the maintenance of a long-term relationship between physician and patient. Several stories describe the sense of privilege at being allowed to participate in the patient's life outside the office.

# HOUSE CALL

*Christopher Dupre*

Dear Mr. C,

As the doctor and I drove to your house for our house call I was quickly briefed on the relevant points of your case in the traditional manner which I was now beginning to accept as the style in which physicians communicate with one another . . . cold, dry, and emotionless. It was also explained to me that you would now be my patient for as long as I was working at the clinic and that today I would handle the entire visit. With a sense of pride I accepted what Dr. M had laid before me and I looked forward to meeting my first patient. As we drove through the woods and finally came upon your small time-weathered trailer I was taken by the pristine beauty of the natural flowers and trees which had grown around it, almost cradling the trailer away from the outside world. As I naïvely entered your trailer it quickly became apparent that nothing so far in my life could have prepared me for what I was about to encounter.

When I first met you, you were sitting up on the side of your twin size bed in the center of the living room clutching onto your weeping wife for support. The only noise in the room was the ear piercing hiss of the green oxygen mask hanging haphazardly from your face. No one in the room dared to say a word. Just as the awkwardness of the moment reached its pinnacle you raised your head and with all the strength you could gather asked me in a quiet and strained whisper—"why won't my heart stop beating so I can just die." As I stood there face-to-face with this once strong and self-reliant man who now looked right through me with his bright yellow eyes that had sunken deep into their sockets all I could reply were three words I feared more than any—"I don't know." Unable to gather my thoughts to form a more coherent and educated sentence I just stood there looking at your emaciated frail body that was draped in a clean white sheet. Your skin was so jaundiced it appeared green in the dimly lit room. In a nearby picture I saw you wore a beard and had thick brown hair which was not all missing after the 12 rounds of cisplatin had burned through your veins. Still unable to think of what to say, I simply sat down next to you on your bed and placed your ice-cold hand in mine. Sitting this close I could hear the strain just breathing was putting on your tiny body. Each breath was becoming more difficult to take and was causing more pain than it was doing good. As we sat there in silence I slowly began to understand, but not accept, what was happening. The welling of water in my eyes must have said it all, and so you, a 62-year-old dying man, gripped my hand and with all your strength you whispered to me the one who was supposed to take care of you— "Don't worry, this is what I want."

As we laid you back in your bed I could see the pain and despair in your eyes as you stared at your wife. As you watched her cry, I could feel the pain you were suffering from seeing her so distraught. Dr. M then put his arm around your wife and told her he thought it might be soon and suggested that this would be a good time to say any good-byes. Sitting next to your bed with your hand in mine it never occurred to me that I would watch you take your last breath, but as we sat there in silence at some point you simply stopped breathing.. There were no alarms sounded or any frantic orders given, just us sitting there hoping you were now in a better place. The calmness of the scene made it almost surreal. As Dr. M placed his hand on my shoulder I could feel the tears welling in my eyes again. When your wife opened the window to let your soul soar out into infinity I felt a tear roll down my cheek . . . I hadn't cried in over 15 years.

I want to thank you Mr. C for allowing me to spend this afternoon with you and your wife and for teaching me about compassion. I truly hope you are in a better place now, because I am for having met you.

♥

# 83-Year-Old Man with Lung Cancer

*Jian F. Ma*

"How are you doing, doctor?" I looked up and saw a tall lanky elderly gentleman smiling at me, probably in his early 70s, wearing a raincoat and a hat with a colorful feather. He was being led into a room by the nurse.

"Thank you, sir, I am fine," I muttered, thinking this is another random small town kindness, and went back to my chart.

Mr. Prince, my next patient is an 83-year-old gentleman with small cell carcinoma of the lung diagnosed 15 months ago. He just had his chemotherapy and radiation therapy and was here for new bilateral hip pain of 10 days duration.

I closed the chart and looked for room 10. Wait a minute, that is the room that gentleman just entered. "I guess he is Mr. Prince." This was the second week of primary care for me and I was still in the inpatient mode, thinking the worst.

I walked into the room and introduced myself:

"My name is Jian and I am a student from Columbia University working with Dr. D today."

"Columbia University? I've seen Columbia doctors before. There was this doctor some 60 years ago who came to Cooperstown and set up the clinic. I still remember that doctor who would make housecalls in the middle of the night. I remember the patient and family would ride a buggy to the doctor's house, or if the patient was too sick, the family would send a messenger to bring the doctor to their house. Do you know how much he charged for a house call like that?"

I know an ER visit at Columbia starts at $275.

"$50." I considered the inflation factor roughly.

"TWO dollars." He smiled. "If the family can't pay for it he would take things like firewood. A lot of the time he gave out medicine for free."

I was amazed by his story. We talked a little more about that Columbia doctor's stories. Now he asked me about the new bone pain he has. He knows he has lung cancer, he can't eat well by himself now and goes to nutrition center once a week. He is steadily losing weight. However, I was surprised to see him having a healthy and younger look. He is such a pleasant man that I really don't want to bring up the possibility of metastasis.

"Mr. Prince, there are a lot of possible explanations for the hip pain. You might have strained yourself or sat in a chair for too long."

"I took some aspirin and that didn't help a bit."

"Well, there is always the spine problem for older people."

"Could it be from my cancer? If it is, how much time do I have?"

"I really don't know without doing some tests." I did the physical exam and not only did he have bilateral hip and spine tenderness but he also has liver tenderness.

"What do you think?"

"I can't draw any conclusion from this exam, it could be a lot of things."

"You can just tell me if it is the spread of my cancer."

"It is the worst possibility, but I can't speculate without more tests. I will discuss with Dr. D and come back to you." I chickened out of the room really quickly. If it is really bad news I don't want to be the one that breaks it.

"OK," Mr. Prince looked disappointed.

I discussed the case with my preceptor and then followed him into the room again.

"Hello, Dr. D, look what I brought you." Mr. Prince's perplexed face suddenly brightened up. He went into his pocket and took out a chocolate candy bar.

"I know you like candy."

Dr. D took the candy and exchanged a few pleasantries with him. Then the patient said:

"Just tell me."

"Most likely metastasis, but we need a bone scan."

"Oh well, I was expecting that. How much time left?"

"Probably months, if it is metastasis."

"I guess I definitely need to finish up a few things."

I could see a hapless expression but he was not totally shocked. Actually he was less disappointed than before. When I was at another clinic I broke bad news to a patient I barely knew. When I told him he had AIDS, he and his family just went berserk and treated me as if I were the one that spread the virus to him. From then on I either avoided breaking devastating news, or, if I have to, I would give a bunch of benign explanations first and hide the most devastating diagnosis in between. I can't really take it when a patient looks into my eye and says "Why?" I guess subconsciously I view this as a failure on my part not to be able to cure the patient. On the other hand the primary care physician, who the patient has seen and trusted for so many years, has nothing to hide. If he wouldn't break the news (good or bad), who would?

"All right, Doctor, thank you for being honest. Eighty-three years is a long time, but its gonna end somehow." Mr. Prince smiled gratefully.

"I wish I could live to your age," Dr. D escorted the patient out of the room.

I watched Mr. Prince walking out to the lobby. If I were the only person working today, Mr. Prince would walk away thinking he just strained his back. Now he walks away prepared and ready to write the final chapter of his story.

♥

# Lung Cancer

*Rose Shorter*

Standing outside the great wooden door, I apprehensively lifted my hand and held it frozen in mid-knocking motion. What was I going to say when I got in there? This was my big chance to do this interview the way I wanted it to be done after weeks of being forced to merely observe my mentors and I certainly did not want to disappoint myself as I tried to execute my plan. I glanced at the chart again, hypertension, diabetes, COPD, an 81-year-old widow. I knew what I would see unveiled behind the door. She would be the standard sweet and demure parched old lady with her large handbag sharing her lap with her displaced and outdated mammary organs. Her cardigan sweater would hang neatly from her shoulders, though the day was warm. She would have translucent curled hair of white or gray, large glasses obscuring her facial features and a sweet and delicate denture smile that she would flash often as she would describe how she is usually so active but just can't seem to get enough energy to wash the dishes anymore.

I relaxed my arm and let it fall to the door with a dull thud, thus accomplishing the cursory knock that is akin to the universal greeting "How are you" without stopping to hear a reply. The knock was immediately followed by my entrance into the room where my gaze landed upon a most unexpected sight.

Sitting regally and straight backed upon the examining table was the most robust and vigorous looking 81-year-old woman that I had ever seen. "Why g'mornin' to ya m'am," she called out to me with a full and rich voice that at once put me at ease and cradled my apprehension in its maternal reassurance. I instantaneously became quite fond of this patient. She had an inviting and friendly look about her while at the same time emitting a no-nonsense and practical air. Her deep blue eyes did not betray her tiredness as they shone and suggested a vitality and beauty long since replaced by the leathery and sun worn skin covering her face and wrinkled into a pattern reminiscent of dry Ramen noodles. The broadness of her face matched the thickness of the rest of her body. Her small and aristocratic nose sat oddly in the middle of this expansive face appearing quite out of place but adding to the majestic bearing of her person.

Taking my seat before her at a considerable height disadvantage, I squinted up at her as the afternoon sun illuminated the back of her head and spilled forth around the edges of her face. As I remembered to begin with my open-ended "What brings you in today?" I glanced down and took note of the hands of a laborer with callused, dry, and cracked skin covering a wide and deep grasp. I wondered how many children had felt the caress of these stern yet nurturing hands. The dirt encrusted under her work worn fingernails gave testament to her refusal to cede to the will of her relentless disease betrayed only by the clubbing of her nails and yellowish discoloration encasing her cuticles.

"I'm really awlright. I was jest down to the barn this mornin' milkin' the cows you know, and m'son, Ted, he told me he wern't gonna let me back till I come here and git miself checked out. I mean I'm fine only I got this chest cold I jest can't seem ta shake."

I proceeded with the usual battery of questions, any runny nose, runny eyes, productive cough, ear pain? Nothing. What next? I rapidly tried to recall what else this chest pain and nonproductive cough could be if not viral or allergic.

"How long has this been going on?"

"Let's see. Al died in October, then, hmm, uh I think 'bout since Thanksgiving."

"That's about five or six months now. Do you have any chest pain, especially when you cough?"

"Well, doc, I sure do. And come ta think of it I sometimes get a little pink stuff up when I cough. But I like tomato juice so it's probaly jest that." She wrinkled up her face in such a way to show that she was not entirely convinced of the tomato juice theory, but she was dogged-ly trying to convince herself that it was true and looking to me for con-firmation of her hypothesis. By this point I had become increasingly suspicious that this was not simply a job for an antihistamine as I was willing to believe before I began questioning her. What next?

"Hmm, how much weight have you lost since November?"

"Well, 'bout 60 pounds altogether, but I ain't had ta exercise much 'cause I sweat so much at night and then I am so thirsty in the day that I drink so much water . . . and tomato juice . . . that I ain't hardly ever hungry. Ted's kinda worried, but I told him I'd jest come and git some medicine for this here chest cold and then I'd git my hunger back."

Now with heightened alarm that I tried not to betray to her, I indi-cated that I would like to move on to the physical exam. Her HEENT was normal. Darn, if only this could be some sort of allergy or flu or even pneumonia. Her heart sounded wonderfully regular. Next I slid my stethoscope to the dreaded part of the exam. Starting high up on her back I asked her to breathe in and out deeply through her mouth. On her first inspiration, she let out a hacking and rattling cough and promptly wiped her hand on the inside thigh of her denim jeans where I could not see the color. When I reached the midway point of her left lung the answer could no longer be denied and dread overtook me. She interrupted my formulations of what to say with, "you know things jest ain't been right since Al died. I mean I'm probably jest sick 'cause I been so sad. But ya know I can't show it ta Ted 'cause he's got his own stuff to deal with."

"I am awfully sorry to hear about your husband. What was it that he died of?"

"Lung cancer."

♥

# Support System

*Mark J. Roggeveen*

He's 75 now and his life is winding down. He knows it, but tries not to think about it too much. It's not that it's been too short, but it just hasn't been long enough yet. This isn't the way that he wanted to go, huffing and puffing when he moves too much with pills trying to wring the blood out of his heart. He has a regimen that's become a full-time job trying to remember and take . . . hydrochlorosomething, and at least four more.

His brother just died last year and he's scared. He's not anxious to join him just yet, at least not this way. Where was the "bang" that he'd always imagined, the heroic last days that he was supposed to have? As a young man, he'd grown up in the World War II era, when men his age were cut out of their prime in numbers too large to imagine. He'd managed to escape it then; he'd survived the bullets and the bombs, now to succumb to his own flesh. It's not that he wants to live like this for much longer, but he just hasn't found a good time to die yet.

Lately, the pills have been giving him some more problems. After he got out of the hospital after his last stay, the doctors changed some of his medicines. Was he supposed to take this one three times a day, or just twice, after meals or before meals? Are there any medications that he could just stop taking? They're expensive, and they're trouble-some to remember to take, but really, they're just a reminder to him that his body is winding down.

"The only pill that we could really get rid of," we told him, "is the antihistamine. Why do you need it, anyway? What are you allergic to?"

"Dogs," he said.

"Are you around dogs often?"

"I have five."

"Hmmmmmmm . . . "

"They like to sleep on the bed with me." A grin crept over his face.

There was a pause, but really, it was all that he needed to say.

We all came to realize that his antihistamine was as essential to his regimen as the diuretic and the ACE inhibitor; and our role was made clear to us. I wished that we could have done more, but we were simply the managers who were trying to keep him alive, trying to eke as many good days out of time for him as possible.

It was his dogs' job to keep him human, to fill those days with purpose. A playful bark, a nip on the heels; they were the meaning in his days. They were the ones that gave him gentle companionship and love.

♥

## Self-Reliance

*Meredith Atkinson*

The couple comes in slowly, because his extreme girth makes pushing her wheelchair clumsy. He won't allow anyone to help though; no one touches the wheelchair but him. In the room, he begins to unbundle her, plucks off her hat, wrestles off her coat. She has extra, disembodied sweater-sleeves pulled on over her arms, an invention I later learn he is quite proud of. Her earmuffs don't come off. Somehow, when I get to the room, he has gotten her propped onto the exam table.

They are late in their sixties, both of them, and it's been a sudden adjustment to helplessness that she has had to make. She has some use of her legs back, thanks to rehab, but now she's at home, and probably as functional as she is going to be. He answers all the questions for her: "I know everything that happens with her every day because I do it all!" He produces a long list of medications on a grubby yellow legal pad, coded into mystifying dosing schedule. He gets frustrated when I can't understand his list, then tries to explain but mispronounces all the names. He tells me to "Look it up! It must be in the records."

"She's helpless, you know. And you know whose fault this is, don't you? But there ain't no use worrying about any of that now. I had to get the car fixed yesterday, and I had to leave her alone for the first time in months. I put her to bed and told her if she had to go, to just go right in the bed. I'd rather clean up later than have her trying to get to the bathroom without me. She hasn't been too hungry, just broth and crackers today. I'm not taking her to therapy today because she doesn't feel well enough." He pronounces it "thurr-apy."

As I approach the patient, he suddenly realizes that he put her pants on backwards this morning, and he is ashamed and frankly apologetic. He tries to fix them until she brushes him away. He hovers during the exam, worried she'll roll off the table, telling me to keep my hand on her at all times. What's more, she seems to play the part of the infant, keeping her eyes closed and letting him respond for her. He says, "She's a real trouper, she is. She's been through so much."

When the exam is completed, he is quick to reapply her layers. As he ties the strings of her knit cap under her chin, he says to no one in particular, "She's my sweety-heart she is . . .I'd do anything for her." He maneuvers her back into the chair, becoming a little breathless in the process. He is dressed like a gas station attendant, and I ask him if he works, but he says he's retired, thank god, and has a 24-hour job with the wife. He says he sees a doctor sometimes, but gets annoyed with all the emphasis on his cholesterol. He doesn't have much concern to waste on himself lately. Overall, talking to doctors is a pretty confusing prospect, and it took a long time for them to let him take her home from the rehab facility, but he knows that she's been better off since them.

He displays no signs of being tired, or discouraged, or resentful. He doesn't sigh or roll his eyes when I remark that he must have his hands full. He doesn't complain that the kids don't come. He wants to share every excruciating detail of their day, but not because he wants me to realize the arduousness of his task. Rather, he wants me to know everything about his wife just in case it might be important, just in case it is a harbinger of a future infection or an indication of a drug interaction. He is single-minded, and his devotion is like another character in the room with us.

Maybe he is so grateful that she's alive that he can't imagine any other way. Maybe he loves her so much that it's easy. Maybe she spent a lot of years taking care of him, or maybe she's always needed taking care of, and this is the course he chose for himself long ago. If he asks for help, maybe that will mean that he's failed, and he thinks his job is to be the only thing she needs. Or maybe, he stays awake at night and worries about being alone and idle, and thinks about how she is all he has, and the only person who would really miss him. And without realizing it, he is doing this to ward off the prospect of a solitary future, and fear gives him the energy to nurture endlessly.

What I begin to see is that he is not unique. He is like another man, so crushed by needing to place his wife in a home that he has sentenced himself to spending 18 hours a day there with her, reintroducing himself to her every morning, eating only institutional food and engaging in no activities. The medications he is given for depression don't help, because he is sad in his soul and they won't reach him there. Or like a woman, who in her late seventies is once again the mother of a three-year-old who used to be her husband, and who lets him follow her around all day and tell her the same story about getting hit by a car over and over. At some point, their spouses can only serve as a reminder that they once lived a different kind of life, that they were loved and had a partner and were not alone. And that must be enough, because they dedicate themselves with a kind of desperate fervor, and they never ask for help.

♥

# Pre-Op

## *David Legro*

"Mrs. V. and her husband are in Room 6. She's having a left mastectomy done next Monday and she's here for a presurgery evaluation. Go on in and talk to her and see how's she doing." I look over her chart: 64-year-old housewife, previously seen only for well-controlled hypertension, biopsy revealed atypical cells, exploratory surgery warranted with mastectomy to look for lymph node metastases, doing well at the time of her oncology appointment last week. She is only the third person with cancer that I've talked to in my life: the first being a patient with metastases to her brain and breasts. These were successfully treated, only to reveal the primary source in her lungs. "I'm taking another trip to Scotland as soon as I get out of the hospital this time," she smiled without tears after telling me that she had decided to forgo any further chemotherapy. I left her room feeling as if I'd been hit over the head. The second was a family friend who was told by his first oncologist that his brain tumor was inoperable and would kill him in six months; the second performed surgery, extracted a mass of cells the size of a baseball, and started him on radiation therapy. Two years later my friend is still working around his house and vacationing in Florida and Chicago, enjoying his retirement in the same way that he did before the cancer was even suspected.

So I walk toward Room 6 nervously. I know little about cancer except that it seems to be ruled so much by chance. One person can be diagnosed with what is called a "good prognostic case" and die from it in months, while others are told they could have as little as a year left to live and still be in good health years later. What will this woman be like? In tears when I enter or calm at first only to break down as I ask her how she is feeling? What can I say to comfort her if this happens? Or will she refuse to acknowledge the possibility of malignancy, even stating that she needs no help? And what about her husband, who may feel powerless to help his wife of many years? Will he be strong or will he need comfort as well?

I knock and enter. She's sitting on the examining table, magazine in hand, her husband reclining slightly in a chair. I introduce myself by rote: "Hello, I'm David Legro. I'm a third-year medical student working with Dr. X. He'll be here to see you in a few minutes; is it all right if I talk to you a little about how you're doing today?"

She has a lined but healthy looking, pleasant face, and she gives me a genuine smile; no strain, no worried look in her eyes. "Sit down, sit down!" she says in an accent I can't place— perhaps German—waving me toward the small chair. I begin by asking if she's here for a check-up before her surgery and she nods. I'm still afraid to discuss the cancer yet, so I start with, "And how have you been feeling since the last time you saw Dr. X?" She feels as she always does, a little tired at times "from my age," but nothing new. She's sleeping well and her appetite is fine; she grins and slaps her stomach while saying this as her husband, a smaller man, laughs.

Before I can bring it up, she does. "So they told you about my cancer?" "A little," I reply, "can you tell me when you found out about it?" We talk about how she found the lump in her left breast while showering three weekends ago; how she had a mammogram and biopsy done the next week and was told that it was potentially malignant but fairly well localized; how she has already met with surgeons and oncologists to plan out her surgery and seven weeks of radiation therapy; and, most important at this time, what she is doing while waiting for next Monday, when she will enter the hospital for her surgery. I ask her if she's keeping busy.

"Well, just as much as he's letting me," she says nodding toward her husband. I soon find out what "keeping busy" means for this couple. They retired almost four years ago, selling their dairy of 100 cows, but "retirement" for them means running three small businesses, including a bed-and-breakfast and selling pies to local stores. They are still maintaining the up-at-4:40 A.M. routine which they began over 40 years ago. This information brings up a flood of anecdotes about their farm, and I'm pleasantly surprised to find myself relaxing, indulging myself by forgetting about the cancer for a few minutes. "Being on a farm is hard work, but it's good for you. When boys came to get our daughters, they had to milk one of the cows before we let them marry them! I think one of them must have s— his pants, he was so nervous, and he never asked for my daughter's hand again!" We all laugh, and I ask if I can listen to her chest for a second.

She is 64 years old, inclining slightly to plumpness, but she has the muscle tone and calluses of someone who has worked hard all her life. I listen to her heart—regular, strong beat, no murmurs, S1 and S2 where they're supposed to be—and her lungs, relieved to find them clear; there are no telltale masses of silence as she takes a breath. Pulses regular. I test her grip strength and she cracks my knuckles in the process. "Hope I'm never in a fight with you," I say, and she breaks out laughing, flexing her right arm.

"Well, you have to be strong in life. That's what got me through everything before, when I broke my arm years ago. They told me not to use it for a long time, but after a few weeks I started using it again." "Much too soon," her husband says, rolling his eyes, and she waves vaguely in his direction. "That's what he kept telling me, but you have to have faith and work for something if you want to get better."

"I think you've got a great attitude about that," I say, and she points at me. "I think that's exactly what you have to have. I ran into a friend in town yesterday, and she starts crying and carrying on, 'Oh, Marge, you've got cancer, oh I'm so sorry!' And I'm looking at her like, 'What's the matter with you? Why are you doing this? Crying isn't going to get me anywhere. You just have to have faith in God and do what you can.' I can't stop the cancer from coming, and if my doctor says I need this operation to get rid of it, I'll do it, but I'm not going to stop doing what I want to do because of it." She says this proudly but gently without a tear or even a pause. There is none of what I was first afraid of here: pure denial. She knows she has a dangerous disease, but while it matters much to her life, she will not let it become her life.

The only "significant finding," for the purposes of the physical exam, that I find is the healing biopsy scar on the upper lateral side of her left breast, still stained with disinfectant after several days. "Have you noticed any other changes? Is your breast sore anywhere?" She shakes her head.

I don't want to leave, but I do after 15 minutes. I report to my preceptor: 64-year-old woman reports for pre-op evaluation prior to left mastectomy . . . I reel off the lack of physical findings and tell him: "They're both really nice. She's got a good attitude."

"She does," he says, and we walk back in. "Still running him ragged?" the doctor asks her, pointing to the husband, who looks skyward in mock despair.

♥

# HOPE

*Sue Cullinane*

We took the office van to Hope, in the North Country, for a home visit. A brief history on the ride included "lung cancer," "real simple people," and refusing Hospice because of a nurse's "attitude." Two miles past Northville, right after the End of the Rainbow Camp sign, go up the dirt path, and it's the green trailer in the back.

The van pulled through the pine trees scattered with trailer homes and rolled to a stop in front of the canned-pea-green trailer. It was this one because of the old station wagon parked by its side. A bounding, barking dog named Brownie met us, offering an easy focus of attention for our entrance.

Mr. O filled the doorway—a sort of St. Nick–looking man wearing an old undershirt over his belly cinched into his green work pants by a belt. Big, thick glasses obscured his eyes. He seemed apprehensively appreciative as we climbed the two steps into the smoke-filled living room. After introductions, he sat at the kitchen table as 'Tricia, the nurse, went off to the back room. I stood awkwardly—tall, and conspicuous in my white coat—trying to somehow apologize silently for my voyeuristic intrusion and 29 years of amassed privilege. Dr. M's warm, booming voice made us all feel more comfortable as he knelt down on one knee to talk with Mr. O eye-to-eye.

The kitchen, a raised continuation of the living room had counters piled with pizza and doughnut boxes, dishes in the sink. On the table, a flyswatter lay ready next to an old cookie tin filled with orange, plastic pill bottles. Mr. O's right hand rested on an ashtray, his fingers stained brown around a lit cigarette. He propped his head with his left arm, covering his mouth with his hand. He pointed toward the new, glossy box of narcotic patches and explained that he would replace the current one tonight, this being the third day.

"But," he said through his fingers, "she's still in pain."

"Are you staying in the bed with her?"

"I've been sleeping on the couch here for the last few, so as not to bother her. She worries me. She only ate a bite of pizza last night and a bite of doughnut this morning." He got quiet, looking askance at Dr. M. "I know when you go, you go, that's it . . . Plans? What do we need a will for? We don't have anything to give anybody but a pile of junk. She's got a bunch of kids, but they don't come round to visit. It hurts her feelings. I don't like to leave her none, except to go down the road when we need some food or pills. I don't want to bring her to the hospital. We been together since she was 21. It's just been us. No, I never seen anyone die in person, in the house like."

He was quiet while Dr. M described death, "a quiet passing in the night, maybe a shudder of the body, no need for pain."

"We don't like to talk about it or think about it much. When it's time to go, she'll go. I'm glad you come, though."

Dr. M rose, saying, "We'll go see her now." 'Tricia came back and sat with Mr. O and we walked back by the worn couch under the window, through a middle room filled with the vibrating whir of the respirator and oxygen tanks. We passed into Mrs. O's room. It was dark and offered only a thin margin around the large bed to walk. Pine-filtered sunlight fell in through high slit windows near the ceiling—casting a dusty haze over Mrs. O, a small figure taking up a sliver of the far side of the bed. She was neatly buttoned up in a faded pink quilted robe, with a lace collar, that reminded me of one my grandmother had worn. Long, silver hair flowed from her head over the pillow; thick eyebrows of the same hue lay above her tiny, crystal-blue eyes sunken under her high cheekbones reined in by her nasal cannula. She folded her delicate, bony hands on the edge of the covers on her chest. She looked ancient and yet childlike—as if the cancer had dissolved years as well as her flesh. Flies hummed and boldly approached her, but seemed to respect her space. Her hand felt tiny and cool in mine as I said, "Hello."

Without movement, she steadily affirmed Dr. M's inquiries as he reviewed her background. She nodded as Dr. M talked about the lovely summer, their spot in the pines, her 86 pounds, shortness of breath, the near frost. We could see and feel the hard tumor pushing out of her rib cage over her left breast. She did not retreat from our pressing hands, but told us of her pain. She smiled at us, and her eyes sparkled. She thought it would be soon. "No, we don't talk about it, we don't think about it. Yes, I'm afraid of pain. I'll go when it's time." She was serene as she spoke and looked at Dr. M, then at me.

In his customary manner, Dr. M turned to me to ask any questions I may have of a woman with lung cancer. I felt my academic enrichment would have to wait for another time. She was a beautiful woman. That's all I could say, and, "Thank you for letting me in." Her eyes captured mine as I held her cool hand good-bye, and the pain in my chest silenced me. Dr. M clenched as well, something I'd never seen him do before.

We retreated and choked cheery good-byes and a "take care now." In the middle room, I asked quick, distracting question about home oxygen respirators to ready ourselves to face Mr. O with strength. He looked up from the table. "It means a lot to us that you come." Dr. M sat down and told him, "It's all right if she goes, or falls when you're not here. You've been wonderful to her. Put on as many of the patches, two or even three, if she feels any pain."

Mr. O clutched his mouth, holding everything in place. A few tears pooled at the rim of his glasses. We stood, held hands, clenched teeth, and fought tears. I was blurred and blinded leaving the trailer. The cool air of the woods helped us make bright good-byes all at once. The now-resting Brownie watched us go. Dr. M, 'Tricia and I walked together to the van, alone in our own thoughts; we waved as Mr. O turned back into the dark doorway. The van crept over the pine needles through the trees leaving the husband and wife their privacy. To say I understood their love, or comprehended their suffering would be self-indulgent and patronizing. I can only say simply—that was an hour in a day that I don't think I'll ever forget.

♥

## HOME VISITS

*Hannah Lipman*

By the eighth and final visit, I wasn't used to it
But I was familiar
A knock on the screen door—then—

Not waiting for a response
(Anticipating, perhaps, when there would be no response)
We'd just walk in

Through the heavy oak door of a beautiful old farmhouse
Or the cookie-cutter metal one in a Senior Center
The same hot moist stale air every time
The smells different, infused with each patient's unique history
But the scene the same

A hospital bed in the living room
Piles of medicine bottles laid out on the kitchen table
Their permanent home
An entire life divided into morn-noon-eve-bed
Like a pillbox
Guided by the visiting nurse, replenishing the drugs
But leaving the morphine in the refrigerator
In the back
Or behind the sugar, available
But not obvious, or enticing

I know that each one has had a whole life
Was a child, a student, a mother, a businessman,
        a farmer, a teacher, a lawyer
Once
They were all different then
But what's striking now are the similarities

A final common pathway of
Hospital smells at home
A kitchen table turned medicine cabinet
And morphine in the fridge

CHAPTER FIVE

# MEMORIES & ANTICIPATION

❤

*O memory, thou bittersweet,— both a joy and a scourge!*

—Germaine Necker de Staël (1766–1817)

Patients and their stories sometimes remind the student of something significant in the student's past. A relative, friend or a situation may be called to mind. Contact with the elderly often evokes a concern for the student's own future and how he or she will face loneliness and dying. The pieces in this section deal with these subjects as well as the lessons learned from patients who have weathered the vicissitudes of life . One student found a parallel between the professional satisfaction of meeting interesting people and the personal joy of becoming engaged to be married during her rotation.

# SINUSITIS

*Eric Michael David*

It happens about once or twice a year, I'd say, and always takes me completely by surprise. I'm usually walking along a very crowded street . . . across Grand Street on a Friday night; down Madison Avenue at rush hour. I see someone with long, curly blonde hair. She has a soft face that I cannot quite make out, but I recognize her posture, her walk, her sense of style. "Meg!" I say to myself. Meg was one of my closest friends, one of those people who watches you grow up just as astutely as you watch them grow up . . . a student of all the changes in your life. She died the summer I turned 21. She had just turned 24. And every time this happens, every time I think I catch a glimpse of Meg on the streets of Manhattan, there is a moment— literally, it can't be more than a tenth of a second—where I think, "Jesus! I have not seen her in ages! I have so, so much to tell her." And that moment is almost as dense with excitement as it is with memories. It is a glorious moment, despite the fact that it ends with the realization, "Well, obviously that is not Meg, because Meg is dead."

J.M. had come to clinic complaining of sinus congestion of two month's duration. Through some great Joycean web of interaction that I will never really understand, primary care clinics seem to have theme days. There was one day where every patient I saw had some urinary tract problem; another day, nothing but foot pain. Today was sinus congestion day, and I was feeling pretty confident with my newly developed therapeutic approach to "doc, my head has been stuffy for months now." I glanced through J.M.'s chart . . . good cholesterol for a man in his mid-fifties. Screening colonoscopy looks great. PSA fine. Generally quite a healthy guy going back through notes from prior visits. A little hypertension, but nothing all our other patients didn't have.

"J.M. is coping much better with his depression following the loss of his son in a car accident last winter," began the next note I came across. I read on: "The boy was in his early twenties, and this was J.M.'s only child. Naturally, he and his wife were devastated, and they have been trying to work through things together. He responded well to an antidepressant." Perhaps the strangest thing about reading transcripts of dictated notes is that, when you have come to know the treating physician somewhat, you can actually hear them speaking the note. J.M.'s physician is a compassionate gentleman with a kind voice. He is a father. I could hear the objectivity in his voice strain as I read.

I walked in and introduced myself. I extended my hand, and we looked at one another for a few moments. It's not that there was anything mystical about J.M.'s eyes. He was, after all, a relatively unremarkable-looking man. Thin. Short black hair with delicate streaks of gray. Brown eyes. Strong jaw resting on his right hand as he sat leaning forward on the examining table. He looked absolutely nothing like Meg's father who had a ponytail and could make a beard look cooler than Jerry Garcia. He certainly looked nothing like Meg's mother. But there was something in the way they all used their eyes.

Meg was one of the first kids I met when we moved to Los Angeles. She went to school with my sister and the two became best friends. My sister was appropriately cruel in the way that one expects a 10-year-old sister to be to a 7-year-old brother. Perhaps slightly more than "appropriately" cruel at times. My sister was also much more extroverted than I, and had made several friends that August when we settled into our new home. I remember tagging after them as they ran into her room one afternoon. I wanted to play whatever it was that was making them all laugh so much, but my sister slammed the door in my face. I remember thinking how the slam of the Los Angeles door was remarkably similar to the slam of the door to my sister's old room in New York. As I walked down the hall to my room, I heard her door open. Meg came running out. She gave me a quick but tight hug and said, "Don't worry, Eric. Your sister loves you." Then she dashed back into the room before anyone could realize she had just comforted the enemy. Who knew a 10-year-old could be so sensitive?

"So let me just make sure I've got everything right," I said to J.M. "You had a cold about two months ago. The sneezing, runny nose, sore throat, and fever went away after about five days, but the sinus congestion has remained ever since that time?" He nodded, then said, "Yes, and I've been using the over-the-counter nasal spray, because it's the only thing that opens me up. But I keep having to use it more and more often. I think I'm getting addicted. Can you get addicted to nasal spray? It seems like a very stupid thing to be addicted to, especially since the relief is so brief." He paused for a moment, and then, "Well, I guess it makes sense. It's those quick pleasures that are always the addictive ones." Although I felt very much engaged in our exchange, I realized J.M. was not necessarily looking at me. His eyes were on the window behind me, where one could look out into the parking lot and a rather busy entranceway to the clinic.

Once, when we were both in college, I went to stay with Meg in her apartment in Greenwich Village. We sat on the floor talking, her immense futon still unassembled in a cardboard box covered in large Japanese letters. The only English words on the box read, "Instructions require some assembly." I pointed to these words and said, "Instructions require some assembly? I guess they give you a set of blank pages and a big bag full of letters."

She looked at me puzzled. I get very serious when people do not laugh at my jokes.

"That was really kind of clever," I offered. "You're supposed to be laughing now."

"I don't get it," she confessed.

"Well, it's the futon, not the instructions, which require the assembly. If we have to assemble the instructions, we're in big trouble."

Meg did not stop laughing for several minutes, then she said, "Why are your jokes always funnier after you explain them? That can't be a good sign. You're lucky you have someone like me who will put up with jokes that require explanation."

I examined J.M.: mild sinus tenderness. No percussive tenderness of the maxillary teeth. Some maxillary sinus opacity to transillumination. Turbinates were unremarkable. Tympanic membranes glistened with the usual bony landmarks. No edema of the eyelids. Pharynx was non-injected. Lungs were clear. I explained that he had a chronic sinusitis, resulting from obstruction to drainage. I told him I thought it would be best to be aggressive and go with a burst and taper of oral steroids.

He transferred his gaze from the window back to me. There was something so familiar about the activity in his eyes. It was the look Meg's parents always have in their eyes, the look my grandmother has had since my uncle died, the look of that couple who lived down the block whose son had drowned when he was six. We talk so much in medicine about facial expressions: the blank stare of Parkinsonism, the haggard, gaunt appearance of hypothyroidism. This look is quite different. It is an awareness . . . almost a kind of scanning. And I am not trying to sound melodramatic, but if you look for it, you will see it in the faces of parents who have lost children. Not always, but I promise you it's out there. It is almost as if they are searching the crowds around them, in wait of those fleeting but profoundly wonderful moments when, just for a fraction of a second, their child is there. That intense flood of excitement and memory . . . a brief but very addictive moment.

After my attending saw J.M., I went back in to explain the course of prednisone. As I spoke, he looked at me quite intently. I was suddenly very aware of his gaze.

" . . . And give us a call in 10 days or so to let us know how your symptoms are. Do you have any questions?"

"How old are you?" he asked. Not a question I was expecting. Was he doubting my clinical judgment?

"Twenty-nine."

"Huh," he said as he rose and extended his hand, "I have a son just about that age, but I don't see him very often." He put on his hat and walked down the hallway back to the waiting room.

# SELF

*Michael Mondress*

I have come to your gray room in the nursing home because the staff says you have, "Not been acting yourself." The chart tells me your history is significant only for progressive dementia. As I futilely poke and prod your unresponsive body in my quest to discover something about you, I wonder what they mean by "not yourself"? Who are you and what can I do to restore your self? I am helplessly staring at your crumpled shell when my attention suddenly shifts to the bulletin board above your head. I see a proud grinning man holding up a prize salmon. One fading picture shows a handsomely dressed man sitting beside a pretty woman. There are four men in uniform standing in front of a World War II bomber. I see laughing grandchildren and I see birthdays and Christmases and seaside vacations. I see family reunions, weddings, and a farm. Even though you cannot communicate, I begin to see the significance of your life. Staring back at you, and then at the snowy scene outside, my reflection becomes more prominent in your window until I am concentrating only on my face. I wonder what lies ahead of me and what my bulletin board will be significant for.

# ON TURNING 27 IN COOPERSTOWN

*Emmy Ludwig*

Mrs. G. is 97 years old. That's 70 years older than I turned, yesterday.
I meet her when I walk into her exam room. I can't see her at first.
The curtain is drawn.
So I ask her if she is hiding from me.
She sits straight up but not too tall on the exam table, wearing
Big blue framed glasses,
    White hair swept up in a lightweight knot,
Achy knees dangling off,
    Ending in little brown shoes.
Somehow, after addressing her knees (oh, they hurt so much in the
    morning),
we're talking about Cooperstown.
Were you born here?
    No, darling, I'm from Canarsie. Brooklyn! Of course I was
    widowed young, at 36. I remarried, eventually. But nothing is
    ever like your first love.
Of course, as ever, I ask for the story.


On this birthday night—it's a full moon—
    After complaining about my advanced age to everyone,
    and talking endlessly on the phone to everyone
    (but feeling a little bit apart from everyone) I treat myself
to a surreptitious much-maligned terribly hypocritical outdoor

cigarette.

Under the truly perfect full moon (made that way just for me, my adoring,
wanted-to-be-a-doctor-too father tells me) I think about the stories I am

collecting.

So how did you meet him?

> Oh, my girlfriend and I went to Coney Island to have a hot dog
> and a ginger ale. We went to a dance hall.

She giggles. I was 17.

> He asked me to dance and then wanted to get my number. But
> I was leaving for the summer so he took his ring off his finger
> and put it on mine, and told me:
>
> > This way I know you'll come back to me.
>
> And I did come back to him. It isn't much but I still have it.

And there on her century-old finger is her husband's ring.

Eighty years after he gave it to her.


Under my moon, I remember that Mrs. G married her dancing partner
and moved with him to this peaceful clear place where I am allowed
to rest for a little while.

Allowed to drink up all the leaves and water and fires and
kindness that I can.

I have no ring. But drenched in the crispy air, besotted by the fall,
and full of stories, I become another year older. It's enough.


Mrs. G is ready to leave. She has a new prescription and a flight to
Florida to catch.

In the last few minutes of her visit she clutches me in a hug.

> I wish I could know you more.

How did you live so long and so well?

> I kept my sense of humor. And God knows best.

Not a bad epigraph, really. I will inscribe it on my moon, in my someday doctor brain, and maybe


consider a trip to Coney Island.

# MOURNING REPORT

*Scott Hummel*

Only one admission last night
Not really very interesting
Eighty some year old gentleman
From Four Fountains
Presented with decreased mental status and
Shortness of breath
(Times
Two
Days)
Let's take a look at the chest films

Nursing home
At the desk
The nurse is busy
She sort of looks up but
Not really and says
"His things are all together
There in the Utility Room."
Eight decades of life somehow shrunken
To half that many shapeless sacks
On the balloon still tied to the walker
(Slightly deflated)
Doctors Mickey and Minnie say
Get Well Soon

As you can see here
The infiltrate had
Progressed

Over the preceding two days
Despite treatment the patient remained
Unresponsive
(Code
Three)
And expired
Shortly
After arrival

Did they know
That he couldn't carry a tune but still
Whistled while he worked
That when you thought
You had him cold in checkers
Five quick jumps
(King me)
Or that every day he wore
White shirt
Dark pants
Dark tie
(Windsor knot)
Except on vacation
Red and black
Hawaiian shirts

Did they know
About the children
And children's children
In one-room schoolhouses
And basketball gyms
And dusty auditoriums
Getting so much more

Than just diplomas
Or that the faith and intelligence
Of his Sunday-school teacher
Inspired him to follow his calling
Or that he loved his family more than
The smell of his rose garden and
The summer sun and
Vanilla ice cream
(Which was a lot)

I say a prayer for them
(And me too)

*In memory of Gus F. Roth*

❤

## JUDGMENT

*K. Ennis Cunningham*

For someone who prides herself on trying not to prejudge others, I'll admit I did not begin my Primary Care rotation in rural upstate New York with high expectations of my patient population. I imagined they might be simpleminded, small-minded small town folks with old-fashioned, uncultured, sheltered, closed minds. It was preemptive hostility. I was worried how they would react to a minority physician, a female who wears her hair naturally. Would they refuse to share their stories? Would they edit their content or refuse to see me? Would they examine me as a novelty item in their examination room like the mysterious mole they might have come in to have excised?

Did that occur? No. Were patients taken aback to have me enter the room? Yes. On one occasion the patient said, "Come on in, son," after being told that a medical student would be coming to see them first. As I came from around the other side of her curtain, she gave a moment's pause. I walked up to her, shook her hand, introduced myself and thanked her for letting me stop by.

"What brings you in today?" I asked. She began slowly with the description of one complaint. As we talked she seemed to relax further and eventually sighed and said, "Well, I wasn't planning to tell you any more but that would hinder your learning process. I've decided to tell you the rest." She began to list all the ways her body had betrayed her and how her life had become overwhelming with the recent death of her daughter from lung cancer. As she began to cry, I sat quietly and listened. I passed her the small box of tissues in the examination room and placed my hand on her lap. When she was finished I briefly examined her and asked if there was anything more she wanted to add before I left to go get her doctor. She said no, paused again. This time without an air of skepticism she looked up at me and said, "Thank you. I really needed that."

During our encounter she implied that she had barriers that she believed would hinder my learning but she wasn't the only one with barriers. It doesn't take a common background to have insight into the sometimes grueling life situations that we will encounter in our offices. If we listen we'll hear people with frustrations, fears of what news the doctor will have, and with stories of the things that bring a light into their eyes—their grandchildren, their volunteer work, their job, their garden. She learned that it didn't require her traditional vision of a doctor for her to leave the doctor's office feeling relieved or better.

Have I felt like a novelty item? Sometimes—I have had patients reach out to touch my hair while I listened to their heartbeat. Yet I wonder if they felt like a novelty as I listened with naïve ears to how many acres they tend and how many head of cattle they milked each morning as I examined their thickened, callused hands. In the city my mind was open to hearing about IV drug use, transsexual operations, and complicated psychosocial histories yet I imagined that a small town would harbor only simple problems and small minds. In the end, it was my small mind that was opened. I hope mine was not the only one.

♥

# EVERYTHING SPARKLES

*Tiffany Holcombe*

"How is your heart, Mrs. R? Has it been giving you any trouble when you walk around?"

She grabs my hand and looks into my eyes with her
sparkling
blue ones.
"My dear, have you ever been to Italy?"

She's not going to answer my question, is my first thought
—maybe she didn't hear it, or is she just avoiding it?

"When we were in Italy, we saw so many beautiful places
—cathedrals, museums
—have you ever been to the Vatican?"

As she talks I look at her shiny,
sparkling,
man's pocketwatch

—it's around her neck,
hanging low,
near her heart.
It's ticking, with perfect rhythm
It was her father's, she tells me
and I wonder if her 83-year-old heart is ticking
just as well.

"You didn't tell me about your heart, Mrs. R—
any trouble?"

"My dear, I was in Italy one month ago
and I saw all of those cathedrals and museums—
I walked to all of them,
up so many stairs,
climbed so many hills
—my heart did just fine."

Mrs. R is just one
there have been so many
—the 92-year-old ex-model
—the man who wore cowboy boots to his stress test
—the old, married couple who are seen in the same examining room
—the man with hearing aids in a leather satchel around his neck
—Mrs. V who wants me to be her doctor when Dr. S retires
—Mrs. T who wants to take me with her to mop her floors
—Mrs. W whose daughter lives in my hometown
—the young man who might have cancer
—the young woman who was in an accident
    and wonders if she'll ever feel normal again
—the pain in the woman's eyes whose mother has Alzheimer's
—Mrs. D, with whom I cried, when she told me how her husband died.

These patients,
who have touched me,
or impressed me,
or both . . .
I think about them
as I walk down the Cooperstown streets each night,
smelling the fireplaces,
crunching the leaves,
hearing the silence,
seeing the stars
and the Christmas lights . . . sparkle.

I'm afraid I've been spoiled
being nestled in this haven—
treated like a doctor,
and loved like a daughter.
How will I feel
when I have to return
to the crowds
to the chaos
to the place that I call home.

But I am lucky, I think
as I look down
at the new
sparkling
diamond
on my finger
— it promises me
that this is not the end of my relationship
with this place,
with these people,

but only the beginning,
and everything around me sparkles.

💜

# They Never Taught Me That

*Joshua Z. Willey*

Bill came in because his friends told him that he had a drinking problem. He had acknowledged it and had come in for help. When I first met him we talked about his drinking, about his past depression, and how his best friend had killed himself, and about what his goals in life were. I recommended counseling or AA and gave him some chlordiazepoxide so he could make it through the withdrawal safely. And all the time I was thinking that there was something oddly familiar about him.

He returned one week later, this time needing some more medication to begin the tapering. He had not found a counselor, but he said he had not been drinking. We talked some more about the importance of the counselor, and I made myself available for anything he needed over the phone. Although he had not seen anyone, I was encouraged by his progress. He left and I thought, perhaps I am making a huge difference in his life. Then, Bill's mother came in 20 minutes later. She was in tears and angry. She accused me of giving him drugs so that he could kill himself. In fact she told me that he was still drinking, taking the medicines, and destroying the family with his talk of hate and death. I consoled her, made sure that she did not feel in danger, and then asked her to bring Bill and any other family members so that we could talk. The anger, sadness, and sense of failure built up, and Bill became even more familiar . . . I was back home. Sitting in the living room with my family around me. We were waiting for my older brother in the room—waiting to confront him. I was scared about the hurtful things that would be said and the risk for violence. I was sad because perhaps I could have been there for him so that he had never taken anything. They told me about glycolysis, gene rearrangements, and the pathophysiology of vasodilatory shock mediated by Acinetobacter sepsis, but they never talked about how patients could remind us of the dark side of our own lives. "Wait, wait, wait . . . you can do this. Be objective, keep your head about you," I told myself as I waited for Bill.

I met Bill and his family. They yelled, they cried, they accused each other of not loving or caring. It was always someone's fault that Bill was drinking. I sat there in silence. I was often not listening—to them at least.

I am back in the living room all over again. "Damn it, clear your head up!" This time mom is yelling: "Do you realize what you are doing to this family?" The reply: "Do you? You taught me this! What kind of mother do these young ones have to look up to?" I yell when the wall gets punched: "Stop this! Can't you see they are crying, why do you always have to yell in front of them . . . " I'm back again when I hear: "Why did he get the medicine?" I answer the question, keeping my scientifically trained mind in it. And yet the memories are there—I continue to relive the whole thing again. I'm failing miserably at this clear analytical mind thing. I have pain, anger, frustration, all directed at my brother for lying, taking drugs, and destroying the family. Bill claims that he is done, that he has hit rockbottom, that he will now quit and seek professional help. My brother said that before he started kicking down doors. I don't believe him, in fact I hate his guts right now. I struggle: "Do you really?" I can't answer that question right now. I resist his pleas in my mind that he is committed to not drinking, that he does not need to be hospitalized. The scientific mind is out the window here; I want to lock him up, I want to punish him. I have been trained though. I give my "I understand," give the impression that I am very empathic for the first time in my life without wholeheartedly feeling the emotion. I know there is something wrong, that I can't stop caring, that I have to think objectively—like a doctor—using the evidence and knowledge that I have. Patients deserve that. I must remember "humanism in medicine," but where was that for me? I struggle to speak, to say something meaningful . . . they never told me about this, never told me how to deal with the fact that I do not know if I am treating Bill or my brother. And I can still hear the screaming and crying of my little brothers torturing my soul, and I too feel like crying all over again. "Stop it—doctors don't cry! What will they think when they see you crying? Professionalism and maturity: fail." I must be the only one going through this—maybe I missed the lecture.

In my head I can't bear it anymore: STOP, STOP, STOP! I cleared my mind just the way I always do when I have bad dreams—the room remains in silence. I wonder how long it has been like that. I remember why I want to be in medicine—to be able to help people in the way that no one helped my family. I focus on Bill and the suffering that he and his family are going through. I ask Bill: "Do you want to kill yourself?" "No, I have never wanted to live more." "Will you see someone to help you today?" "Yes, I know I need the help, I want to stop drinking." I ask the mother and brother: "Are you all willing to help? Do you understand that he has a disease and that he needs you to support him and not stop doing so even when he relapses? This is harder to treat than cancer or any other disease you can think of. He must do this with help from his family—that is the only cure." "Yes, we understand the pain that Bill is going through, and he needs our help. Bill, allow us to help you." "I will mom, I know I can't do this shit anymore." The room becomes warm again as they embrace. I no longer hear the screaming. I make myself available for anything that they need, and they are off to see the counselor. I pray that they are able to understand the nature of this disease quickly—it took me only six years to do the same for my brother.

I leave the room after them, in good spirits, with a seemingly renewed sense of hope that they, and I, can do this. I sigh because I am relieved and exhausted. I feel like I just got off the spinning ride at the carnival. I present the case to my preceptor like I do any other case. I give my assessment and plan, but I cannot talk about what was going through my mind. How could he understand?

I go home and watch TV for the rest of the day, staring blankly into the screen, my mind blank . . . it needs a break. I must be a terrible student to let my emotions get in the way of the care I provide. This is not even the first time it happened. I felt inadequate in trying to help Bill. I wish they told me how to deal with this stuff before. I may never see a patient with lymphomatoid granulomatosis, but I've read about it and they have tested me extensively about it. And yet Bill is the second similar case; that other time with the 50 year-old suicidal woman . . . that was rough. I must be the only one who gets this stuff.

They have taught me about removing preconceptions and biases, to use counter-transference, and rather vaguely about taking care of yourself. I learned a valuable lesson from Bill. They could have never taught me that. But then again, perhaps they knew that no one could do it better than Bill. I'll never know. Regardless Bill and his family will always be on my mind, and I pray we meet again someday. I think they'll make it. I'm not sure what Bill would say to me, but I know that the first words out of my mouth will be "Thank you."

♥

# Remembering the Golden Tiger

*April Zhu*

My grandmother passed away years ago, and my grandfather left us in January 1999. Qing Niang means grandmother. Ye Ye means grandfather. After all these years, some words still seem dearer to me when spoken in Chinese.

My grandparents had lived in the same house on the outskirts of Shanghai for more than half a century. When they first moved in, all of the houses were new and the neighborhood was designed for young professionals. After the Communist liberation in 1949, the population boomed and housing became unavailable. As my aunts and uncles married, walls went up, vertically and horizontally, to accommodate the new family members. Spacious rooms where kids once played ping-pong became claustrophobically subdivided. My grandparents' room upstairs, however, was spared of having an attic put in. I still remember staring up at the high ceiling and humming fan on those distant hot afternoons when I was forced to take naps.

My grandparents' room was full of wondrous things. On the walls hung fading black-and-white portraits of ancestors mostly unknown to me. In one of those photos a slender young woman stood in a field of tall sunflowers, her pretty face in profile. Qing Niang was 19 years old, and Ye Ye was the amateur photographer. She wore a traditional dress with a stiff high collar. Her hair was in the fashion of a time before the Japanese and the Communists—when Shanghai was still the Pearl of the Orient.

On top of his enormous and ornate desk, Ye Ye kept a collection of calligraphy brushes. Some were as thick as my arm and others as fine as a fountain pen. The brushes were well worn, the handles stained with ink, and filled the room with a familiar scent. By the time I got to know Ye Ye, he was a well-respected scholar and calligrapher. He had long retired from engineering railroads that reach far into the outer provinces. On the precious few weekends I was able to spend with him, starting at age four, Ye Ye began to teach me calligraphy. Though I didn't know many characters then, he had me copy poems in the styles of ancient masters. At times, Ye Ye stood over me, his powerful hand over my timid one, and showed me the subtle nuances of handling the brush. A swoop, a pause, a flight—the brush as agile as a bird. The cigarette in his other hand enveloped us in translucent swirls of smoke. The mingling of calligraphy ink and cigarette smoke is as potent for me as the madelines were for Proust.

I loved looking through Ye Ye's drawers when no adults were around. Scattered among the mundane papers were curiously heavy coins from the time of emperors, stone stamps with artistic carvings of Ye Ye's name, and thumbnail sized photos of infant grandchildren. One of the small side drawers contained an assortment of hardware. Oddly shaped scales and cryptic slide rules, cheap plastic cigarette lighters and handsome steel engraved ones. Satin gift boxes holding brushes of rare animal hairs, presented to Ye Ye by admiring younger artists, were thrown into yet another drawer and dismissed as showy materialism.

Ye Ye had an elaborate nian tai, a piece of stoneware upon which calligraphers tapered their brushes and meditatively rubbed ink sticks with water to make the black liquid. An uncle had gone a considerable distance to purchase it from a region known for that type of stone. Despite the traditions of calligraphy, Ye Ye was an impatient man. He used store-bought ink, pouring it into a glass cylindrical cigarette container. He tapered his brush on the side of the glass and left the nian tai as an ornamental piece.

For his cigarettes, Ye Ye didn't use a proper ashtray either. His was a stout bronze container that sat on four delicate dragon's feet. I was frightened as a child when I was told that the container was intended to hold incense for the dead. The underside of the urn was stamped in an antiquated script that I couldn't read. The urn had been in the family for a long time, Ye Ye remembered his grandfather using it too. It must be from several dynasties ago.

Ye Ye was born in the year of the Tiger. He loved the tiger motif. When I first moved to Los Angeles from Shanghai, I remember buying him a 1987 calendar with pictures of tigers. Many years later, when Ye Ye visited us in Salt Lake City, he found a small golden statue of a tiger at a yard sale. He wanted me to have it. We are the most powerful and fanciful symbols of the zodiac, he liked to say, the aging tiger and the youthful dragon. Ye Ye liked his golden tiger so much that didn't want to leave it behind when he returned to Shanghai, so he told me to bring it back to the States after he dies. I hate talk of death.

A healthy octogenarian, Ye Ye had better energy and sharper mentation than some of his children. He practiced calligraphy every morning and read classic texts in the afternoons. He was active in the city government as well as in artists' associations. He composed poetry, worked on his autobiography, and still found time to e-mail. He spoke with great enthusiasm about coming to America again to attend my medical school graduation.

Both of his older brothers lived healthful lives well into their nineties, despite having smoked heavily from a young age. Ye Ye recalled visiting one of them before his death. The brother was unable to speak, but when they were alone, he held up his index and middle fingers. Ye Ye understood and took out a cigarette. His brother held the unlit cigarette to his nose and smiled. Ye Ye dismissed advice to quit smoking. "I'm too old to get cancer" was his inevitable retort.

I returned to China two months before medical school was to begin. We started our trip in Beijing, where Ye Ye and several relatives met my mother and me. The weather was unseasonably hot for early June, and Ye Ye was of low energy and spirits. When we arrived at the bottom of the Great Wall, he was already exhausted by the comfortable car trip and refused even to ride the cable car to the top. An old Chinese adage dictates that to be a true hero, a man must climb the Great Wall. Ye Ye had been there several times already, this time he waited at the foot of the mountain. Throughout the two weeks in the Beijing, Ye Ye complained endlessly. The air conditioning in the car was uncomfortable and the hotel mattress intolerable. He wanted to have the best Peking Duck in town, but then sat through the decadent evening eating only one piece. Everyone was anxious to go back to Shanghai.

At home, Ye Ye returned to his routine. He continued to practice in the morning, but allowed me some time on his desk to practice as well. Humbly, I must reveal that I was Ye Ye's favorite grandchild. I was the only one who studied calligraphy seriously, and I won numerous competitions. I stopped practicing, however, when I went to America. Once again at the enormous and ornate desk, my brush was more like a turkey: surely Ye Ye was hiding disappointment when he told me my childhood foundation was still evident. He encouraged me to practice regularly again. It clears the mind and cultivates the spirit, he instructed. Indeed, calligraphy served as meditation for him, but at other times he continued to be disagreeable.

Shanghai summers are unbearably hot and humid. Some afternoons, even the cicadas stop singing. Neighbors, mindful of electricity costs, fan themselves outside, sitting in bamboo chairs under tree shades. In Ye Ye's room, a silent battle took place over the air conditioner. I, the extravagant and pampered foreigner, liked the temperature at 26°C. Ye Ye kept adjusting it to 31°C. He complained of stiffness and bone pains and blamed the air conditioning for being too artificial and too cold. His favorite, and therefore the most insolent, I argued with him. I thought he was trying to save money on electricity. Decades of war, famine, and revolution have made thrift a way of life for his generation. I dismissed his complaints.

Weeks went by, but Ye Ye's fatigue and pains continued. He became less animated. His afternoon naps became longer, he lost interest in his books, and he ate less. I tried harder to entertain him.

I asked him to tell me stories from his life and the history of the Middle Kingdom. I took him on walks and urged him to play chess with men from the neighborhood. From the city center, I brought home his favorite foods and new pajamas. For his eighty-fourth birthday, I bought him a glossy calligraphy book and we browsed it together. I did manage to amuse him a little with a cigarette lighter I gave him. The lighter looked exactly like a cigarette, and he teased visitors with it. But overall, Ye Ye remained unchanged. Finally, we went to the hospital.

Ye Ye first decided to go to an orthopedist. They suggested a traditionalist and prescribed a Band-Aid brand skin patch containing a chili pepper ingredient. On another floor of the hospital, the traditionalist advised some analgesic herbs and acupuncture. Ye Ye was not the sort of man who believed in herbal remedies or acupuncture. He was rarely sick and dismissed most bodily complaints as hypochondriacal. His theory was that the body heals itself, and that the doctor serves only to comfort the person. Ye Ye continued to blame the air conditioning and I backed down.

Time passed quickly. It was soon time for me to leave Shanghai. As I stepped into the taxi, Ye Ye held my hand tightly and told me this was our final parting. Don't be ridiculous I told him, my vision becoming blurry, you have to come to graduation.

A few months into my first year at medical school, Ye Ye was diagnosed with lung cancer. I don't know the type, grade or stage, and I didn't know to ask back then. The odds had beaten him, the cancer had spread to the bones. Ye Ye was sent home to be cared for by his children, and they sat by him every hour of every day. My mother rushed home to Shanghai, while I stayed at school. The winter was unusually bitter, and, despite the coal and electric heaters, the old house couldn't be heated enough. My mother began knitting furiously, racing against time, as if the anger and force could be directed at the metastasis. Ye

Ye protested, saying he won't live to wear it. My aunts were touched and picked up the needles while my mother slept.

They described to me the final days. Ye Ye screamed and cried in pain. He was frustrated that he was too sick to kill himself and insisted to his children that he wasn't a weak man. When I was young, Ye Ye told me stories of how he lived in a shack on the Gobi desert, suffered hepatitis during the famine, and endured attacks from Red Guards in the upheaval. He ate onion and garlic raw. I never questioned his strength. Late in his disease, some friends secured illegal opium and it was made into a tonic. Surely if Ye Ye's mind was clear then, he would have told his children that opium is to be smoked. When the delirium fully set in, he wrongly accused the family of hurtful deeds. In his mind, he distorted me into a wicked grandchild and believed that my gift of the glossy calligraphy book was really cheap promotional material distributed by a museum. When he died, seven months after our trip to the Great Wall, Ye Ye weighed less than 50 kilograms. The sweater was too big. I am glad I never saw him that way. I will always remember him as engineer, poet, artist, teacher, hero, and my most devoted fan.

Ye Ye's ashes are buried next to Qing Niang, on a quiet mountain overlooking a bay. It's an appropriately tranquil retreat for a scholar, one that is often depicted in the Chinese paintings that he liked. The old house will be torn down soon to make room for new highways. My relatives are moving to further suburbs. Shanghai is undergoing unprecedented growth and renewal.

I can only imagine what they will find in the crevices of that house. The detritus and treasures tell our history. I've written to my relatives, asking them to find my golden tiger. I will go back when I graduate. I will kneel at the grave and burn incense in that bronze urn from several dynasties ago.

# CHAPTER SIX

# FINAL IMPRESSIONS

♥

*Where there is love of man, there is also love of the art.*

—Hippocrates (*Precepts*)

The students' academic experiences during their first primary care exposures vary in some respects—some make house calls, others don't; some work with one physician, others work with several. But it is neither the diseases encountered nor the setting in which the visits occur that define this seminal period of training. It is the demonstration that whatever the disease, and whatever the seriousness of it, the skills of communication and caring are important both diagnostically and therapeutically. Bassett adds a social dimension to the experience because of the rural and small town environment. The final piece in our collection provides one student's reflection on the details and overall significance of her time in this unique place. We would like to think that the lessons she learned are typical of all who venture into primary care. We hope that, like her, students leave this and similar programs aware of the importance and satisfactions of getting to know patients. It is good to see that patients and the learning experience make "a lasting impression."

# A Lasting Impression:
## What I Learned in Cooperstown

*Ann Salerno*

I learned what primary doctors do.
I learned to ask the right questions.
I learned to listen to stories.
I learned that everyone has a story.

I learned that history is king.
I learned that people like a doctor who smiles.
I learned that doctor really does mean teacher.
I learned to appreciate the amazing opportunity I have to be entrusted
   with the lives of others.

I learned that a smiling 66-year-old woman with Down Syndrome
   can really brighten your day.
I learned that 70-year-olds can act like 16-year-olds when they are in
   love.
I learned that 91-year-olds can sometimes look better than 61-year-olds.
I learned that it's important that elderly folks be independent.

I learned to allay the fears of little old ladies.
I learned to treat the low back pain of big young men.
I learned that most people don't get admitted.
I learned that no one wants to be in the hospital at Christmastime.

I learned about farmers.
I learned that cows get mighty angry when they are thirsty,
and that they may push you down and break your bones.
I learned that people get really excited about hunting.

I learned that the big city isn't the only place to see great medicine.

I learned that little hospitals can make a big difference.

I learned that great nurses are key.

I learned that there actually are a lot of people who do take their medications.

I learned that sticking 10 medical students in a big old house in a small town for a month can be great fun.

I learned to share the bathroom and one phone.

I learned that a Christmas tree can brighten up an old house with ugly furniture.

I learned that you can get really cool Christmas gifts from people you just met.

I learned that doctors spend as much time with people as they do with paper.

I learned to press pause less often while dictating.

I learned that insurance companies are a pain in the butt.

I learned that Medicare doesn't care.

I learned that losing your wallet is a huge pain, but not the end of the world.

I learned that small town store owners will go out of their way for their customers.

I learned how to change my car battery.

I learned that the supermarket is the place to be on a Friday night.

I learned that it snows a lot more on the other side of the Catskill mountains.

I learned that you never grow out of sledding.

I learned that baseball was invented in Cooperstown.

I learned that sewing machines were a good idea.

I learned that there are a lot of people who are depressed.

I learned that there are a lot of people with hypertension and high cholesterol.

I learned about PMR.

I learned that smoking is really bad.


I learned that you don't have to remember every drug we learned in pharmacology class.

I learned that you don't have to do a stress test on everyone with chest pain.

I learned that some people will never stop talking if you let them continue.

I learned that doctors get great desserts from their patients.


I learned that my career choices are unlimited.

I learned that doctors can have time to do cool stuff like bike and hike.

I learned that I don't want to live in a town where everything closes at five o'clock.

I learned that I do want to live in a town where the doctors go to the high school play.


I learned that doctors have the coolest job in the world.

I learned that seeing patients is very tiring.

I learned that this job is right for me.

I learned that behind each exam room door, there sits a new experience—a person to learn from, a person to teach, a person who has the opportunity to leave a lasting impression.

# Afterword

♥

## About the Mary Imogene Bassett Hospital

The Mary Imogene Bassett Hospital in Cooperstown, New York, operates a system of clinics and hospitals (collectively known as Bassett Healthcare) serving an eight-county region of central New York State. Named for a remarkable physician who died in 1922, the organization was established more than 70 years ago by a group of idealistic young physicians and surgeons as a salaried group practice combining patient care and teaching in a rural area. A formal academic association with Columbia University College of Physicians & Surgeons was established in 1947.

Active training programs for some 50 resident physicians in internal medicine and surgery ensure a stimulating academic atmosphere for physicians, allied professionals, and students. Research has been part of Bassett's mission since its beginning. Social and scientific ventures developed at Bassett include an early successful pre-paid community health insurance program and seminal research in bone marrow transplantation by Nobel Prize winner Dr. E. Donnall Thomas.

Humanism in medicine has always been at the heart of Bassett's training and practice. Attracted by this tradition, as well as by excellent technical training, senior students from Columbia and other schools have come for inpatient and subspecialty clinic experience for over 50 years. As recognition grew for the need for specific training in the skills of general primary care medicine, in 1989 the University of Rochester asked Bassett to participate in Rochester's innovative "Medical Practice Based" experience for third-year students. In 1992 Columbia created a similar requirement. Some 30 to 40 students a year now benefit from the highly sought-after experience at Bassett in the offices of general internists and family physicians.

In 1999, a formal program in Humanities and Medicine, based on original proposals by Drs. Alan Kozak and Michael Foltzer, was established at Bassett as an outgrowth of the successful student-writing project. The program was awarded a National Endowment for the Humanities Consultation Grant in 2000 to facilitate development of a dialogue between physicians and the public with the goal of improving understanding and communication. The primary aim of the various activities of the Humanities and Medicine program remains the support of Bassett's tradition of training caring health professionals.

# Reading List

♥

*Literature and Medicine* is a semiannual scholarly journal published by the Johns Hopkins University Press.

Many medical journals include occasional creative writing, historical vignettes, photographs, and articles pertaining to the humanities.

Journals that frequently offer creative writing and papers addressing the role of literature in medicine include:

*Annals of Internal Medicine*
*Journal of the American Medical Association*
*Academic Medicine*
*Health Affairs*

# NOTES